EUROPEAN-AMERICAN ELDERLY
A GUIDE FOR PRACTICE

Christopher L. Hayes, Ph.D., is currently Assistant Professor in the Department of Psychology at Long Island University, Southampton, NY. He was formerly Director of the Center for the Study of Pre-Retirement and Aging at The Catholic University of America. He completed his B.A. and M.A. in clinical psychology at Duquesne University and his Ph.D. at the Fielding Institute of Santa Barbara, California, in human development with a specialization in gerontological services. His major areas of interest include ethnic/minority aging and clinical/practice issues in working with the elderly.

Richard A. Kalish, Ph.D., is self-employed as a writer, researcher, teacher, and consultant. He completed his B.A. at Antioch College, his M.A. at the University of Maryland, and his doctorate at Case Western Reserve University, all in psychology. He has published more than 130 journal articles, book reviews, and chapters in books. He has also written or edited 14 books. Almost all of his academic work has dealt with issues relating to aging, death, and loss of loved ones.

David Guttmann, D.S.W., is Associate Professor and Chairman of the Master's Program at the National Catholic School of Social Service (NCSSS), The Catholic University of America (CUA). He received his doctorate from CUA in 1974. Formerly he served as Director of the CUA Center for the Study of Pre-Retirement and Aging and as Assistant Dean for Academic Affairs of NCSSS. Noted for his research in gerontology, Dr. Guttmann is the author of many publications on aging.

EUROPEAN-AMERICAN ELDERLY

A GUIDE FOR PRACTICE

Christopher L. Hayes, Ph.D.

Richard A. Kalish, Ph.D.

David Guttmann, D.S.W.

Editors

SPRINGER PUBLISHING COMPANY
New York

Springer Publishing Company, Inc.
536 Broadway
New York, NY 10012

86 87 88 89 90 / 5 4 3 2 1

Library of Congress Cataloging-in-Publication Data

European-American elderly.

   Bibliography: p.
   Includes index.
   1. European American aged. 2. European American aged—Services for. 3. Social work with the aged—United States. I. Hayes, Christopher L. II. Kalish, Richard A. III. Guttmann, David.
HQ1064.U5E85   1986   362.6   86-11878
ISBN 0-8261-5450-6

Printed in the United States of America

This publication was produced under Grant No. 90AM0104/01 from the Administration on Aging, United States Department of Health and Human Services, Washington, D.C.
   The findings, opinions, and conclusions expressed in this publication are solely those of the authors and do not necessarily reflect nor can be inferred as being the official position or policy of the Administration on Aging.

CONTENTS

CONTRIBUTORS

James J. Burr, M.S.W., is currently Scholar-in-Residence at the National Association of Social Workers in Silver Spring, Maryland. He completed his B.A. at Holy Cross College, Worcester, Massachusetts, and his M.S.W. at Boston College School of Social Work. He is a member of the Gerontological Society of America, National Association of Social Workers, Academy of Certified Social Workers, and the American Public Welfare Association.

Michael A. Creedon, D.S.W., is the Virginia Prentice Andrews Professor of Gerontology at the University of Bridgeport in Connecticut. He was formerly Director of the Center for the Study of Pre-Retirement and Aging and assistant professor in the National Catholic School of Social Service (NCSSS) at The Catholic University of America. He completed his M.S.W. at Virginia Commonwealth University and his doctorate in social welfare at the University of Maryland (Baltimore) with a specialization in gerontology. He was previously head of Social Development for the Southern Virginia region of the Roman Catholic Diocese of Richmond, Virginia.

Donald E. Gelfand, Ph.D., is a Professor in the School of Social Work and Community Planning of the University of Maryland and the author of *Ethnicity and Aging.* He has been a Senior Fulbright Research Fellow in the Federal Republic of Germany and a Senior Research Associate at the National Council on the Aging. Currently he is serving as secretary of the Social Research, Planning, and Practice Section of the Gerontological Society of America.

Joseph Giordano, M.S.W., is presently Director of the Center on Ethnicity, Behavior, and Communications for the American Jewish Committee. He has done pioneering work in integrating ethnocultural factors into mental health practice, and his articles have appeared nationwide in papers and magazines. He is a co-author of *Ethnicity and Family Therapy.*

Zev Harel, Ph.D., is Professor of Social Services and Director of the Center on Applied Gerontological Research at Cleveland State University, Ohio. He completed his M.S.W. at the University of Michigan and his doctorate at Washington University, St. Louis. He is a consultant, advisor to planning and service agencies in the field of aging, and member/officer of numerous organizations in the field of gerontology.

Che-Fu Lee, Ph.D., is presently Director of the Center for the Study of Youth Development and Associate Professor of Sociology at The Catholic University of America. He completed his M.S.W. at Oklahoma State University and his doctorate at the University of North Carolina (Chapel Hill). He is a member of the Gerontological Society of America, the Population Society of America, and the American Sociological Association.

Irving M. Levine, B.S., is currently Director of National Affairs and Director of the Institute for American Pluralism at the American Jewish Committee. He received his B.S. from New York University (NYU) and has done graduate work at NYU's Center of Human Relations as well as at the School of Social Work of the University of Wisconsin.

Terrence G. Wiley, M.A., teaches linguistics and English as a Foreign Language at California State University at Long Beach. He is also pursuing his doctorate in curriculum instruction, with a specialization in multicultural education, at the University of Southern California. He has co-authored two textbooks on second language acquisition. He is a member of the organization of Teachers of English to Speakers of Other Languages and the California State Association of Teachers of English to Speakers of Other Languages.

PREFACE

Since the early 1700s the United States has opened its shores to immigrants who seek a better way of life. With the recent influx of refugees from southeast Asia and various Third World countries we have once again recognized that we live in a very pluralistic society characterized by individuals of different ethnic and racial backgrounds. Today there are thousands of elderly Americans born in Europe who are 65 years of age or older and who speak a language other than English in their daily communications. This group, which is often referred to as *Euro-American elderly,* played a significant role in fueling this country's industrial expansion despite limited education and a lack of English-language fluency.

Traditionally, Euro-Americans relied heavily on their family, ethnic organization, and church or synagogue for assistance in times of crisis. However, due to the mobility and shrinking size of the family and to changes occurring within ethnic urban neighborhoods, this assistance is no longer as readily available. In addition, many of the younger family members are less willing or able to continue to provide culturally expected assistance to their aging parents due to marital, child-rearing, or employment responsibilities. As with the older adult population in general, the Euro-American elderly are living longer and will need more formal and informal supports in dealing with age-related problems.

In every major city in the United States there are large ethnic enclaves where thousands of limited-English-speaking elderly live. Increasingly, the suburbs are also home to the Euro-American elderly. Common to all of these elderly people sooner or later is a need for assistance—public, private, or a combination of both. The majority of these people do not benefit from available services because their cultural values often prevent them from admitting a need and, consequently, from seeking assistance. There are others, however, who probably would use older adult services if they knew how to obtain them.

Unfortunately, as research has shown, they often do not know that these resources exist or how they can apply for them. Euro-Americans would benefit greatly if accurate and relevant information were made available to them about the public services to which they are entitled as taxpaying American citizens. They also need to know about programs and services in the private sector that may be helpful to them.

This book is the result of a variety of historic efforts that were critical in bringing the concerns and issues of the Euro-American elderly to the surface. The pioneer research effort of Dr. David Guttmann in conducting the 1979 Administration on Aging grant entitled "Informal and Formal Support Systems and Their Effect on the Lives of the Elderly in Selected Ethnic Groups" laid the foundation for understanding the cultural patterns of behavior, values, and attitudes of Euro-American elderly. Most important, this research indicated the necessity of evaluating ethnic factors in planning services for the aged. A more extensive discussion of this work and the impetus it provided for the 1980 White House Mini-Conference on Euro-American Elderly can be found in Chapter 1.

In 1984 the Administration on Aging funded a second grant, entitled "Facilitating Family and Community Supports for the Euro-American Elderly with Language Barriers," under the direction of this author, who continued the effort to assist this group. A major activity of this grant involved conducting a National Conference on the Euro-American elderly held at The Catholic University of America in May 1985. The conference assembled ethnic leaders, policymakers, and service providers. Its mission was to increase our understanding of the ways that the Euro-American elderly can obtain better access to services and benefits that are available for older adults. The knowledge generated from that conference is reflected in the various chapters of this volume.

This book attempts to guide the reader to information, program strategies, and service models that will be helpful in working with the Euro-American elderly and their families. To address this purpose, the content is divided into three major sections. Part I presents the sociocultural background of the Euro-American elderly and includes a variety of historical and developmental perspectives that are critical in understanding the world view of this group. Part II discusses social institutions, such as the family network and the ethnic neighborhood, that play central roles in the lives of the Euro-American elderly and are important factors in the provision of services. Part III concludes the book and identifies a number of intervention strategies, program models, and research efforts that enhance the well-being of Euro-American elderly. More important, this section provides potentially valuable guidelines for the development of new culturally appropriate services for this aged subgroup.

Any organization or professional person engaged in delivering human services to the elderly, especially those whose work brings them into contact with the ethnic aged, will find this document useful. It is hoped that the background information and practical insights within this publication will motivate decision-makers, both within and outside the ethnic community, to more fully address the needs of the Euro-American elderly.

A recognized danger in developing a book of this type is to encompass all nationalities from central, eastern, and southern Europe under one banner. Because of space and resource limitations it is impossible to reflect the diverse language, cultural, and religious differences inherent in all of these different groups. Where possible, every attempt is made to be sensitive to the importance of making cultural distinctions. It should also be noted that many of the ideas discussed are applicable to other minority groups who have strong ethnic identification and similar language problems.

The foundation of this effort is the recognition that the Euro-American elderly represent a valuable asset to this country. The varying customs and traditions that they brought from foreign lands have enriched the fabric of America. Now that they are older, we must continue to recognize them as a unique group with specific needs and perspectives. It is my hope, along with the other editors, that this book is a positive step toward this endeavor.

Christopher L. Hayes, Ph.D.

ACKNOWLEDGMENTS

The editors wish to express their utmost appreciation to Barbara W. Stone of the Center for the Study of Pre-Retirement and Aging at The Catholic University of America. Without her patience and word processing and editing talents this publication could not have been produced. In addition, the editors wish to thank Pauline Mahon-Stetson, Andrew Hofer, and Joann E. Smith for assisting with the technical aspects of coordinating the grant that produced this document. Finally, we would like to thank the Administration on Aging for funding Grant No. 90AM0104/01, "Facilitating Family and Community Supports for the Euro-American Elderly."

PART I:
Sociocultural Background

1

A Perspective on Euro-American Elderly

David Guttmann, D.S.W.

> "I had turned away from my Jewishness," said Runya
> Schwab, 74 years old. "I married a militant atheist, and I
> considered myself to be more Socialist than anything
> else." Subsequently she recalled, "I was divorced and
> found myself without friends. So I needed to seek out
> people with whom I could relate, and I automatically
> sought out Jews. It was a reawakening process." (quoted
> in the *New York Times*, 1985)

Almost 60 years ago, on May 6, 1926, a more famous Jew's letter
was read to the Society of B'nai Brith. The occasion was his 70th
birthday, and Sigmund Freud wrote:

> That you were Jews could only be agreeable to me; for I was myself a Jew, and
> it had always seemed to me not only unworthy but positively senseless to deny
> the fact. What bound me to Jewry was (I am ashamed to admit) neither faith
> nor national pride . . . but plenty of other things to make the attraction of Jewry
> and Jews irresistible—*many obscure emotional forces,* which were the more
> powerful the less they could be expressed in words, as well as a clear con-
> sciousness of inner identity, the safe privacy of a common mental construction.
> (Quoted in Erikson, 1968, pp. 20–21).

In a recent conference on Euro-American Elderly held May
17–18, 1985, at The Catholic University of America a story was
told of an old woman in a nursing home. She was placed there as

someone without a family or relatives and was given up as hopeless by the staff, who thought her to be deaf and mute. But one day a visitor spoke to another person in a foreign language. Then, to the astonishment of the staff, the old lady who was thought to be deaf and mute started to speak fluently—in her native language.

What is common to all of these stories is the discovery of that mysterious and powerful element in human life—namely, ethnicity—which, however ignored or suppressed, comes back to haunt us as we advance in years. Ethnicity means relating to a community of physical and mental traits in races, or designating groups of races of mankind discriminated on the basis of common customs and characters (Webster, 1948). Ethnicity, in general, is expressed chiefly through attitudes and values commonly held by a group of people and by a sense of a common core or a historically derived cultural uniqueness that binds people together with a sense of identity.

Each ethnic group has developed over the centuries its unique patterns of aging and its own attitudes toward the aged. These significantly influence individual perceptions of old age—whether as a time of joy, wisdom, and continuity of social involvement or a time of despair, destitution, and depression.

In this chapter an attempt is made to review the situation of the Euro-American elderly from a historical/theoretical perspective. Attention will be paid to issues of (a) composition and diversity, (b) immigration and coping patterns, (c) concerns and interests affecting well-being, and (d) explanation of the concept of social networks that help Euro-American elderly cope with stress. The purpose of this presentation is to show

- Who are the Euro-American elderly?
- How did they come to the attention of policymakers in aging?
- What are their chief problems?
- What strengths do they possess that could be used by leaders and service providers alike to serve those who need social services?

WHO ARE THE EURO-AMERICAN ELDERLY?

Our definition encompasses all ethnic people of European origin—both old and new immigrants, prior to or after World War II. This broadening of the term *Euro-American* is based on the 1971

TABLE 1.1 Euro-Ethnics* as a Percentage of the Population, by Sex, 1972

	TOTAL	MALE	FEMALE
All Ages Population			
Number (000)	204,840	99,378	105,462
Percent	100	48.5	51.5
Euro-Ethnics			
Number	63,428	31,054	32,376
Percent	100	49.0	51.0
Non-Euro-Ethnic**			
Number	141,411	68,323	73,088
Percent	100	48.3	51.7
Euro-Ethnics as a % of population	31.0	31.3	30.7
65 and Over Population			
Number	20,146	8,262	11,884
Percent	100	41.0	59.0
Euro-Ethnics			
Number	7,079	2,917	4,162
Percent	100	41.2	58.8
Non-Euro-Ethnics**			
Number	13,067	5,345	7,722
Percent	100	40.9	59.1
65 and Over as a % of Total Population			
Population	9.7	8.3	11.3
Euro-Ethnic	11.2	9.4	12.9
Non-Euro-Ethnic	9.2	7.8	10.6

*German, Italian, Irish, French, Polish, Russian.
**Includes not reported.
Source: U.S. Department of Commerce, Bureau of the Census, *Characteristics of the Population by Ethnic Origin,* March 1971 and 1972.

and 1972 count of the United States Census as indicated in Table 1.1.

Taking this 1972 census as a base, we see that more than 7 million Euro-American elderly comprise the 65-and-over population, who are the subject of this book. This sizable proportion of the total elderly population of the United States reflects more than the six ethnic groups referred to in Table 1.1. In fact, Euro-

American elderly consist, in alphabetical order, of Albanians, Armenians, Basques, Belgians, Bulgarians, Byelorussians, Carpatho-Ruthenians, Croatians, Cypriots, Czechoslovaks, Danes, Dutch, Estonians, Finns, French, Germans, Greeks, Hungarians, Italians, Jews, Latvians, Lithuanians, Luxembourgers, Maltese, Norwegians, Poles, Portuguese, Romanians, Russians, Serbians, Slovaks, Slovenians, Spanish, Swedish, Ukrainians, and Yugoslavs. One could also add the English, Irish, Welsh, and Scots, as these ethnic groups also originate in Europe. However, they are not usually included in this designation because English is the common language.

Not only are ethnic groups different from each other, they also have a differential use of cultural and social resources. For example, eastern European and American-born-and-raised Jewish elderly differ significantly in their leisuretime activity interests because of different backgrounds and culturally conditioned preferences for meaningful and enjoyable activities. While they certainly share a common sense of peoplehood, ancient history, and positive attitudes toward Jewish values, they may differ rather sharply in the social networks they utilize. They also differ in use of language (Yiddish vs. English) and especially in their participation in social club and voluntary associations (Guttmann, 1973).

Lopata (1976), in an excellent presentation entitled *Polish Americans* and subtitled *Status in an Ethnic Community,* shows the differences in the availability of social networks between numbers of the old and new Polish-American immigrants. She cites the classification of several types of societies that are involved in the life of the ethnic community:

1. The tribal society, designated by a distinct name, united by a belief in common ancestors from which culture was originally derived, and possessed of some degree of social integration.
2. The political society, which has a common legal system and an organized, independent government controlling all of the people who inhabit a definite territory.
3. The ecclesiastical society, which has a common and distinct literary, religious culture and an independent, organized church.
4. The national culture society, which has a common and distinct secular, literary culture and an independent organization functioning for the preservation, growth, and expansion of this culture.

Each of these societies consisted of a social network of organizations so that members, if they desired, could limit their significant interactions to its confines. Lopata (1976) states:

> Members of the old emigration have village and regional idealities in common. New emigration Poles share common experiences of displacement. Each group identifies differently with Poland, America, and Polonia. Other important variables distinguishing one Polish American from another include generations in America, occupation, age, sex, marital and parental status, education, and presence or absence of an extended kinship group. These traits affect a Polish American's (1) social class lifestyle; (2) involvement in Polish, Polonia, and American variations of this lifestyle; and (3) content of life. (pp. 4–6)

The Euro-American elderly represent much more than a silent majority among the minority groups of the aged in American society. These people with their heavily accented English are the ones who, along with all other elderly, have spent a lifetime of effort to make this country strong, affluent, and free. These are the people who, along with others, worked hard to build neighborhoods and cities; fought in many wars; made major contributions to the cultural, artistic, and scientific life of the country; and enriched the general welfare of society. They are also the people whose needs, wishes, concerns, and worries are seldom heard.

Yet a lack of political assertiveness on their part does not correspond to a lack of interest in their own welfare. Nor does it indicate a lack of expectations on their part about a wholesome and meaningful existence in old age. Rather, it is a result, perhaps, of the assimilationist pressures of the past—to become American, to *melt,* and to shed their cultural heritage—which have intimidated them and undermined their belief in the legitimacy of their cultural values.

The Euro-American elderly were not represented in the White House Conferences on Aging prior to 1981. This lack of representation was due largely to the inability of this group to organize themselves into a political entity as the Black, Hispanic, Asian, and Native American elderly have. They failed to utilize political pressure for recognition and legitimacy by the federal government.

The process whereby the Euro-American elderly became visible among the various minorities within the aging population has barely begun. Its early traces were rooted in the work that was invested in the President's Commission on Mental Health held in 1978. Volume 3 of the report of that commission dealt with special populations and has for the first time recognized "Americans of Euro-Ethnic Origin" as a separate entity among minorities.

In 1979 another milestone occurred. The United States Civil Rights Commission held hearings specifically on Euro-Americans. This was a historical opportunity to raise in a public forum the various problems besetting them and to open up, with the representatives of the government, dialogue concerning ways and means to ensure the well-being of Euro-American elderly. However, the 1981 White House Conference on Aging (WHCOA), along with its Mini-Conferences, was the vehicle that finally pushed the Euro-American elderly into the limelight.

The idea of convening a special White House Mini-Conference on Aging for Euro-American Elderly originated with this author and was recognized by the executive director of the 1981 WHCOA. Undertaken as a joint project with the National Center for Urban Ethnic Affairs, it was supported with funds and encouragement by the National Endowment for the Humanities and by ACTION. The two mini-conferences held subsequently in Baltimore (November 10–12, 1980) and Cleveland (December 4–6, 1980), constituted the best vehicles for enabling elderly Euro-Americans to participate in the mainstream of society. Each conference involved approximately 200 people; and voting delegates consisted of representatives of national ethnic organizations, local and neighborhood ethnic organizations, and individual leaders of Euro-American elderly. The two White House Mini-Conferences on Euro-American elderly were the first historical events to bring together ethnic elderly and their representatives from many different Euro-American communities, with government, public, and private sector participation.

The recommendations that resulted from the 1981 White House Mini-Conferences on Euro-American elderly clearly established what government's role should be in assisting the Euro-American older population. Of primary concern was the contention that the government has not recognized the Euro-American elderly as an identifiable and distinct group that includes resources and strengths that can be effectively employed to overcome barriers to service delivery. Mini-Conference participants saw government as not recognizing that many Euro-American elderly do not receive their fair share of services and benefits to which they are entitled. Of the many specific recommendations made in the *Report of the Mini-Conference on Euro-American Elderly,* the following are of special interest in this book:

- The Euro-American older population should be clearly recognized by all levels of government as an identifiable group in the older population and one whose various social, spiritual, and economic needs and strengths should be recognized in both the programming and the policymaking process.
- Residents of ethnic communities, especially the elderly and their organizations, should be formally involved in all private and public policy decisions involving service and resource allocations affecting their neighborhoods.
- Any outreach program aimed at the older population, particularly with regard to various major public social programs, must have appropriate and effective ways of reaching and informing the older Euro-American population.
- Wherever there are concentrations of older Americans with limited English-speaking ability, bilingual staff who are fluent in the ethnic languages of the elderly should be available to serve as liaisons and facilitators between the formal and informal support services that serve the elderly.

How did all of this come about? For an answer we will look at further background information on the Euro-American elderly.

IMMIGRATION AND COPING WITH THE NEW LIFE

A nation of immigrants, the United States has absorbed well over 50 million newcomers from all corners of the world, comprising more than 100 ethnic groups, about 50 of them major groups. The main influx of immigrants occurred in two periods: the first, also called the *old immigration,* deriving mainly from northwestern Europe and lasting from about the 1830s to the 1880s, involved more than 18 million immigrants; and the second, called the *new immigration,* lasting from the 1880s until World War I (or 1914), involved more than 23 million immigrants, mainly from east and south Europe. (President's Commission on Mental Health, 1978).

The saga of the immigrants and their struggle with the harsh conditions of the "promised land" has been told and retold in countless books, plays, poems, and musical and artistic creations, as well as movies and television shows. The endless fascination with this theme attests to the heroic proportions of human endurance, perseverance, and faith.

The time of arrival of immigrants to the United States and the attitude of society at that time toward newcomers are important variants in the adjustment of immigrants in general and, consequently, also in the outlook of ethnic elderly. The present Euro-American elderly, especially those of eastern and southern European origin, came not only from different cultures, but even if from the same cultures, by waves at different times. These waves, sometimes generations apart, left their country at different historical periods. Thus, they often had radically different experiences of being raised under the rule of foreign powers or in periods of their country's independence and freedom.

In some groups—for example, Polish, Slovak, Hungarian, and others—there are still some elderly who arrived in the United States before or shortly after World War I, although most of their elderly were born in the United States. In these ethnic groups there are also elderly who belong to the post-World War II immigration; and some, such as Estonian and Latvian, count most or all of their elderly in this relatively recent immigration. It is easy to understand why these elderly would have different social, cultural, and emotional problems from those who arrived two generations earlier. It can also be expected that most of the later arrivals may still have some language problems and consequently may avoid contact with the general community and its service agencies.

The typical immigrant family, settling during the mid- to late 19th century, was primarily engaged in rebuilding its ethnic culture and, through a distinctive socialization process, in creating new generations in the image of the old (Mindel & Habenstein, 1976). They were kin-involved and community-situated, and they generated neighborhoods that combined to form urban villages (Gans, 1962). Threats to the family, whether perceived or real, contributed to in-group solidarity.

The early ethnic family was large, with nuclear units embedded in households of extended kin. Three generations under the same roof was the norm. Families were unified through division of labor, habituated role-playing, family rituals, ceremonies, and group participation in both sacred and pragmatic activities. With their systems of mutual and reciprocal aid, families were structured to remain viable in this world of strangers and external institutions. They remained insular and resistant to the network of institutions and voluntary associations that form a social structure for an industrial society with its impersonal market economy (Mindel & Habenstein, 1976).

For ethnic groups the family remained a primary unit of social organization and a source of identity bound by strong affection and loyalty. Once transplanted, the immigrant family maintained its adult-centered character and its place for the elderly, who contributed as long as they could and helped to perpetuate the cultural heritage of the group.

With the rapid industrialization and urbanization in the past century came an increase in geographical and social mobility, changes in the family and kinship system, and changes in the socioeconomic situation. Consequently, the cohesiveness of the ethnic community and the traditional support systems to the ethnic elderly began to crumble. There was the flight of the younger generations to the suburbs, while the elderly remained and tried to hold onto properties earned in a lifetime of hard work. The physical separation of the elderly from their children and grandchildren put family relations under great stress. The telephone and automobile could not replace the intimate, if not always ideal, intergenerational bond. The ethnic communities, having lost their most dynamic members, stagnated and slowly disintegrated. Parishes were abandoned or changed hands (Kolm, 1977).

Each ethnic group coped with its problems in its own peculiar way as dictated by its culture and its historical experiences. Some did try to relocate their communal resources with all of the institutional patterns of relationship and function, but their main efforts focused on the young—the only hope of the survival of their ethnic identity. The community left the elderly either to depend on their families or to find their own resources. It is certainly true that federal support in the form of Social Security and Supplemental Security Income (SSI) and local support through low-cost public housing have aided the elderly financially. However, the same financial supports that have enabled the elderly to live independently may have harmed some individuals in a way not anticipated by social planners. The elderly person who lives alone may suffer severe loneliness, particularly at a time in life when physical mobility is decreasing and contacts with family and friends become ever more difficult to maintain.

CONCERN AND INTEREST IN EURO-AMERICAN ELDERLY

Concern about and interest in the ethnic aged are of very recent origin. While general gerontology grew rapidly after World War II, serious discussion of the ethnic factor in aging began only in the last few years. However, social scientists, especially anthropologists, were aware of the cultural differentiation in the developmental process long ago. Erikson's (1963) theory of life stages in psychology and Parsons' (1968) study interrelating personality with cultural and structural patterns in sociology made significant contributions to the subject by relating cultural differentiation to modern societies and modern man.

In the past, members of Euro-American groups have often failed to utilize mental health services (Giordano, 1973; Giordano & Giordano, 1976; Struening, Rabkin, & Peck, 1970). This is probably related to two salient facts: values related to self-sufficiency and a lack of accessible services. Self-sufficiency means not only being able to provide financially for one's family but also being able to take care of one's own personal problems. When such problems occur, members of these groups have had to rely traditionally on primary associations—ethnic groups, family, extended family, religious organizations, or neighborhood associations—as opposed to professional services. Today there are signs of change in many ethnic communities. While it is true that a tradition of self-sufficiency still remains as a buffer against mental illness, an overromanticization of how well cultural resources function has led to the myth that Euro-Americans do not need nor seek out professional services.

The toll of living in our society and the weakening of those intermediate institutions—family, ethnic group, religion, neighborhood—that have traditionally acted as buffers to stress are reflected increasingly in a rising demand by Euro-Americans who are seeking professional help to solve their emotional and family problems. These people share many of the problems of other ethnic groups. However, it should be emphasized that each group has its own cultural patterns and its own diversity that makes it unique (President's Commission, 1978).

In most Old World cultures the indigenous, traditional support systems to the aged, such as the family and stable community patterns, were and still are very much in operation and taken for granted. On the other hand, in New World heterogeneous cultures such as the United States, the impetus toward assimilation has been a serious deterring factor in the development of interest in cultural differentiation. As a result, it took the pressures of such social issues in the United States as the War on Poverty, the racial revolution, and, finally, the resurgence of ethnicity to open the way to considerations of cultural factors in aging (Kolm, 1977).

The traditional support systems—the family, the stable residential neighborhood, and the parish for Roman Catholic groups—

remained the chief, if not the only, support systems of the ethnic aged for at least two generations. Some innovations did, however, occur during that time. Under the impact of the larger society, new support systems such as the mutual-help fraternity and the community hall were added. Both, however, remained within the boundaries of the ethnic community and retained a personalized character in relation to members of the community.

The main issues in the welfare of Euro-American elderly concern the particular support systems, informal and formal, still existing in the various American ethnic groups and the relationship of such supports to the efforts of society in general to alleviate the problems of its aged. In the traditional society they provided an in-group support to the nuclear and extended family. These included friendship groups and the special organizations—churches, voluntary associations, and so forth—that were concerned with helping the aged to cope. In contrast, the modern communal framework includes both the larger community and the subcommunities, such as neighborhoods and ethnic groups.

As people age, their circle of significant others changes. For most elderly people there is a narrowing of the number of friends and confidants available as resistance resources to stress. Issues in social network research concerning ethnic minority elderly are complex. How do they engage and involve themselves in acquiring new people to serve as significant others within their social context? How do they go about enlarging their social worlds or life spaces? How do older people differ in utilizing to the fullest their life spaces, which include the areas of social interaction around which people organize their behavior, the physical environment of home and familiar possessions, and the psychological environment of roles and status within the community? Life space makes up the assumptive world. Changes in any of its areas, whether positive (achievement or gain) or negative (loss), signify transition. Since life space is part of us, these changes raise anxiety and lead to stress, which, in turn, necessitate activation of resistance resources; restructuring of our thoughts, feelings, values, and actions; and coping with new situations.

SOCIAL NETWORKS AS RESISTANCE RESOURCES TO STRESS

Network utilization can teach us about the aged person's ability to cope with stress and about the availability and responsiveness of network (family) members, whose emotional attachment and filial obligations lead to the provision of care. In this light, it is surprising that very little research has been done on the differences among various ethnic minorities in dealing with stress experienced by their aged members.

Perhaps the most common source of stress is decreased economic resources. Among all races, elderly women are the hardest hit by poverty, while of all poor persons 7 of 10 men aged 65 years and older live in poverty (Rowan, 1981).

What causes the difference between pathological and nonpathological response to stress? Why do substantial numbers of subjects who live under similar conditions (e.g., poverty, ignorance) not become ill? The answer to both questions is resistance resources, which are defined by Antonowsky (1979) as the power that can be applied to resolve a tension expressive of a state of disturbed homeostasis. The rapidity and the completeness with which problems are resolved and tension dissipated are central elements of tension management that can be applied to the social–emotional functioning of individuals and groups.

There are three major social–psychological resources available in varying degrees to the individual dealing with stress. The first is homeostatic flexibility, or the ability to accept alternatives relative to (a) social roles (for example, accepting alternatives to employment); (b) values (for example, accepting values other than your own as legitimate); and (c) personal behavior (for example, overcoming personality conflicts in a work situation).

The second major resistance resource to stress is ties to others, which focuses on connections people have outside their families, such as close friends.

Finally, the third major resistance resource to stress, called ties to the community, involves the nature of people's relationships within their communities, including the frequency of their interaction and involvement with community members and functions as well as their perceptions of the status and power available to them.

It must also be recognized that there are some dysfunctional factors involved in ethnicity. Ethnocentrism, withdrawal, clannishness, social rigidity, prejudice, and tendency toward intergroup conflict are all well-known dysfunctional aspects. However, as with individuals and interpersonal relations, situational factors such as societal pressures for social and cultural conformity are inevitably at the root of these dysfunctional aspects of ethnicity and ethnic diversity in society. A solution to these dysfunctional aspects of ethnicity is not eradication of cultural differences but the development of their best potential. Although the question of the general desirability of cultural pluralism cannot be answered unequivocally, it can be assumed on the basis of historical experience and recent research that it can be superior to homogeneous cultures regarding social integration, cultural productivity, and even political strength (Kolm, 1973).

CONCLUSION

Today, overall, there is greater awareness and acceptance of ethnic diversity in American society. The roots phenomenon is more than romanticism of the past. It is a sense of peoplehood; it is a searching to find new ways of better understanding and to draw on those supports that help people to cope more adequately with adaptation and daily stress (President's Commission on Mental Health, 1978).

Euro-American elderly have made their "debut" on the stage. How well they will play their roles with respect to innovative ideas about self-help, self-reliance, community cohesion and support, intergenerational relationships, and continued contributions to the welfare of all elderly people in this society remains to be seen. The President's Commission on Mental Health, the U.S. Civil Rights Commission Hearings, and the 1981 White House Conference on Aging served their purpose in highlighting the issues that concern Euro-American elderly. However, the response must encompass each and every ethnic community in which Euro-American elderly reside.

2

The Meanings of Ethnicity

Richard A. Kalish, Ph.D.

Ethnicity is a living reality, a way of life, a source of enhanced well-being and belonging. These words, modified from an informal note written by one of the experts on Euro-American elderly, express the other side of the coin. The more familiar side of the coin is inscribed with ethnicity as a *problem* and as a characteristic that one must live with and try to relate to positively.

The side of the coin that we want to represent in this chapter is ethnicity as part of one's self, so totally integrated into the self that the self can no more exist apart from ethnicity than apart from gender or age. The emphasis of the past three decades has been on the ethnicity of Blacks, Hispanics, Asian and Pacific Basin groups, and Native Americans. This has occurred with good, historical reason. However, the personal meaning of ethnicity for members of these groups is, to the best of our knowledge, no greater than it is for members of what we are describing as Euro-Americans or, for this volume in particular, Euro-American elderly.

VIEWING ETHNICITY

Ethnicity can be viewed from the outside as a characteristic attributed to a given individual on the basis of which the viewer makes certain assumptions about that person. Ethnicity can be viewed from the inside as a basis for group identification and belonging. One authoritative source offers 14 characteristics that underlie ethnicity, although no one ethnic group is likely to encompass all of the characteristics. These are geographical origin; migratory status; race; language or dialect; religious ties or faith; ties through kinship, neighborhood, and community; shared traditions, values, and symbols; literature, folklore, music, and so forth; food preferences; settlement and employment patterns; special interests in regard to politics in the homeland and in the United States; institutions that specifically serve and maintain the group; an internal sense of distinctiveness; and an external perception of distinctiveness (Thernstrom, Orlov, & Handlin, 1980). These are not to be seen as equal in importance for either a particular individual or an ethnic group. Rather, they may be viewed as guidelines.

This author has integrated what he sees as the most significant features of the various approaches to ethnicity and has developed the following explanation of the concept: Ethnicity refers to (a) group membership based on (b) the integration of (c) values and feelings and (d) practices and behavior that (e) arise through historical roots in the family of origin and (f) through common cultural, religious, national, and/or linguistic background, and (g) culminate in a shared symbol system and (h) a sense of shared identity. This approach suggests that ethnicity is a living reality, a way of life.

Writings about the Euro-American elderly have tended to focus on those from eastern and southern European nations, with less emphasis on immigrants from northern and western Europe. The work of Guttmann et al. (1979a) is representative of this emphasis. Two probable reasons can be outlined: first, those who immigrated here from Europe during the past 100 years have been disproportionately from southern and eastern Europe; and second, these ethnic groups have remained more visible than groups from the north and west of Europe. All in all, from the 1880s to the beginning of World War I, some 23 million immigrants arrived from Europe, most of them from eastern and southern Europe (Kolm, 1980). Although some did return, most remained here, had their families, grew old, and died here.

Overall, however, there is very little information about Euro-American elderly. For the most part, they are subsumed as part of the population designated White or Anglo, without any recognition that this very large grouping of individuals is extremely heterogeneous. When differentiating Euro-ethnic data are provided, an additional complication enters: the divisions are often based on national origin rather than ethnicity itself. Therefore, a category such as "East European/Soviet Union" brings together persons from Poland, Russia, and the Ukraine, some 17% of whom are Jews. To combine the first three groups means combining fairly distinct ethnicities; including the Jews adds a fourth distinct ethnicity. While these groups undoubtedly share certain characteristics, Glazer (1984) represents those who believe that conclusions based on this kind of combined data base can be misleading.

INFLUENCES OF ETHNICITY ON THE INDIVIDUAL

Ethnicity and ethnic-group membership influence the individual in many ways, ranging from food preferences, to skin color, to political influence. In a previous study this author has outlined four ways in which ethnicity can affect the individual members of the ethnic community (Kalish, 1983).

First, people outside the ethnic community react to individuals in part in terms of their ethnic membership. Likes and dislikes, expectations, and stereotypes maintained regarding the ethnic group are frequently applied to the individuals within the group. Sometimes these views are based on personal experiences, although even personal experiences are screened through prior beliefs and expectations. Sometimes the views are largely or completely the result of early socialization and values learned through the family and community and having relatively little relationship to actual experiences.

Second, individuals who are part of the ethnic community respond differently to other members of their own community than to persons outside the community.

Third, expectations and perceptions of self are influenced by ethnic-group membership. The success or failure of each member of the ethnic community can be viewed as reflecting back on the individual.

Fourth, ethnicity has a direct influence; that is, each of us will be a little different from others not of our ethnic group in terms of values, speech, manners, history, role expectations, family relationships, and so forth.

When Euro-American elderly are considered in terms of these four approaches, it quickly becomes obvious that the elderly are also affected by their age-group status in the same ways that members of the ethnic community are affected by ethnic-group status: the non-elderly react to older people in terms of their age;

other older people also respond differently to the elderly than to non-elderly; expectations and perceptions of self are affected by being elderly; and being elderly has a direct influence on behavior.

To understand older European Americans, then, it is necessary to understand (a) older people and the aging process, (b) Euro-American communities, and (c) older people within Euro-American communities.

SUBGROUP AND INDIVIDUAL DIFFERENCES

Within every ethnic group there are innumerable subgroups, and within every subgroup there are innumerable individuals, all of whom are unique and few or none of whom are precise fits for the modal characteristics of the group. Thus, in viewing Euro-American elderly, we constantly need to keep in mind that the larger the unit (that is, Euro-American elderly versus Croatian or Greek elderly versus those Ukrainian elderly living in the Logan area of Philadelphia), the greater will be the heterogeneity of the individuals within the unit. There will be greater within-group variability among Euro-American elderly in general than among elderly Croatians or Greek Americans in general, and greater variability among the latter groupings than among the elderly Ukrainian Americans living in the Logan area of Philadelphia. However, even among the latter, there are still considerable individual differences.

Among the bases for subgroup differences are education, occupation, region of the homeland from which the older person came, region of the United States in which the older person settled, the density of the ethnic population where the older person resides, and the nature of the local ethnic community. The bases for individual differences include all of the unique qualities that lead to individual differences among any group of people: early socialization, family and particularly parent–child interaction, early experiences, adult socialization and experiences, and many other factors.

The glass may be seen as half full or half empty. We can focus on the cohesiveness within an ethnic community and among Euro-American communities or on the schisms; on what binds the individuals together or on what keeps them apart. What impresses this author most is that these ethnic communities, in spite of differences within and between, have maintained a strong sense of identity for over a century. Although undoubtedly the form has altered over the decades, the customs, rituals, language, values, and a sense of group belongingness have continued; and this occurs even though the members often leave the original neighborhood, become diverse in terms of careers and education, and develop close friendships and working relationships outside the ethnic community.

AGE COHORT AND IMMIGRATION COHORT

An *age cohort* consists of those individuals who were born and therefore reared during the same approximate time period. An *immigration cohort*, a term not generally used although the concept is familiar, consists of those persons who arrived in the United States at approximately the same time. In understanding today's Euro-American elderly, we need to be concerned with both age and immigration cohorts. Being part of the same cohort means that certain experiences are shared at the same age, which presumably will intensify the sense of sharing.

For example, all persons conscious of baseball in the 1930s were aware of the DiMaggio brothers. Those who were born in the United States between the end of World War I and the "crash" of 1929 could be considered an age cohort; they were all made aware of the DiMaggios at approximately the same age. Today they constitute the young-old generation. Those who are also ethnically Italian may well have shared a personal sense of satisfaction concerning Joe, Dom, and Vince that age peers of other ethnic groups did not have. Further, when recent Italian immigrants arrived here, Joe DiMaggio was already baseball history, and Dom and Vince were almost forgotten. Therefore, the later arrivals, although of the same ethnicity and possibly the same age cohort, were of a different immigration cohort and did not experience as youngsters the feats of the DiMaggios. If we replace the baseball example with the example of responses to the role of Italy in World War II, the importance of knowing both age and immigration cohorts may become more apparent.

As each immigrant group comes to the United States, it seems to face one common major conflict: the extent to which the individuals should maintain the values, customs, behavior, and identification that they brought with them from their homelands versus the extent to which they should adopt American ways of doing things. As time goes on, new generations born in the United

States increasingly tend to impose on the ethnic community their ideas as to appropriate functioning, usually in the direction of greater acculturation and assimilation. Nonetheless, at times younger generations appear to be in the vanguard of those wishing for a revival of ethnic customs and values. At the same time, more recent immigrants from the homelands arrive, usually under different conditions than the initial arrivals, and make their impact felt on the ethnic scenes.

The elderly are part of each of these groups: the immigrants, second- and third-generation, and recent arrivals. Understandably, for the most part, they are more likely to be heavily represented among immigrant and first- and second-generation Americans than among very recent arrivals or later generations (we are referring here to Euro-American elderly, since other ethnic groups have different patterns).

The immigration cohort that arrived in this country between the 1880s and the beginning of World War I is now all elderly. By the time another decade has passed, only a relative handful of survivors, all well into their 80s, will still be alive. Yet only a decade ago these individuals were in many ways the dominant age-and-immigration cohort of the Euro-American elderly. This points up the need for more accurate information so that we can improve our knowledge as to what, in fact, is taking place with the Euro-American elderly because it is obvious that changes are occurring and, further, that these changes vary considerably across individual ethnic communities. (Che-Fu Lee's chapter on demography in this volume offers an excellent beginning for such understanding.)

HISTORY IN THE UNITED STATES

When this nation was established, some 80% of the white population had British ancestry (Gleason, 1980). As is understandable for a new nation, there was immediate concern with developing an American nationhood and nationality. The assumption was made that those of non-British background, at least those who were neither Native American nor Black, would blend with the British-origin majority into one nationality. Ethnic diversity was viewed "not so much [as] an essential feature of the national identity, as a condition that America transformed in the process of creating a new nationality" (Gleason, 1980, p. 33).

As each new immigration wave arrived, beginning in the 1830s and ending only with the advent of World War I, it was greeted with immediate pressure to drop the old ways and become Americanized. At the same time, the new arrivals had various reasons to maintain the values, rituals, and behavior that they brought with them from their homelands. When the numbers of immigrants became sufficiently large, conflicts were engendered between the immigrant groups and those Americans who viewed themselves as in the mainstream. These conflicts led to job and neighborhood discrimination, stereotyping, and sometimes violence. Newspaper editorials and politicians frequently inveighed against the immigrants.

In 1908 playwright Israel Zangwill's *The Melting Pot* opened on Broadway to great acclaim. The theme of the play was that the various ethnic groups in the United States, limited at the time to those of European origin, were like different metals that, when placed in a heated pot, would melt down and combine, emerging as one strong, durable, beautiful metal with characteristics of its own. The term *melting pot* subsequently became identified as representing the position that not simply acculturation but assimilation would eventuate in the greatest value, both for individuals and for the United States as a nation.

This author recalls from his childhood in the 1930s the stories told by his father and family friends of their own conflicts between the desire to respond to the pressures felt in the schools to become good Americans, which meant to become assimilated, or the wish to maintain their loyalties and express devotion to their parents and ethnic communities. Some had once viewed their parents as "greenies" or greenhorns, newcomers who did not sufficiently take on the values, practices, and everyday behavior of what was then mainstream America. The older generation was once seen as looking back, both in time and in terms of their country or culture of origin, while the new generation saw itself as looking ahead to a unified, modern America.

Such recollections of this author represented the melting pot philosophy. However, in spite of those who actively pursued this approach and the pressures that others felt to do so, for the most part these people—those who became teenagers and young adults in time to fight World War I and to suffer from the Depression of the 1930s—retained their loyalty to their parents and a strong sense of identity with their ethnic community. Even as early as the 1920s, the melting pot philosophy came under attack, and its history for the past 80 years has been a series of fights between its supporters and its detractors. The acceptance it received at one time was replaced by rejection of its tenets a decade or two later.

As the melting pot and assimilation faded from being the dominant approach, acculturation became accepted, with its support of accommodation to the larger society and functioning effectively within it but without losing the positive aspects of ethnic identity. Favor now seems to be shown to cultural pluralism or the acceptance of numerous cultures that function side by side in some contexts and retain their individual uniquenesses in other contexts.

Assimilation implies that diversity has a negative valence. The new pluralism proposes that diversity is a sign of strength. It encourages individuals to benefit from the positive attributes of their ethnic community—the sense of belonging to a supportive group, the link to one's historic past, a feeling of connectedness to people who live in other places and who lived in other times so that one is not alone in the universe—without feeling that this diminishes in any way their loyalty to the United States as a nation.

Many Euro-American elderly lived through the period when the melting pot view was at its strongest. The public schools and the media denigrated their ethnic values, practices, and identifications. But even the most casual survey of the past 80 years will show that whatever support the melting pot philosophy might have had among writers, educators, and policymakers, it made only modest headway among the individuals to be influenced by it. Certainly, large numbers of European immigrants, their children, and their grandchildren did become highly acculturated and even assimilated, but enough maintained ethnic identity so that many Euro-American communities are still visible and viable today.

Younger age cohorts and more recent immigration cohorts did not experience the power of the melting pot philosophy, but most Euro-American elderly have experienced its effects. This could result, at least for some, in reluctance to offer a public display of ethnic values or in shame at an inability to use English effectively. It might also make it difficult for some to accept the more aggressive actions by Blacks, Hispanics, and others because such actions appear to violate the values promoted by the melting pot approach that dominated their introduction to appropriate behavior in America. This might also explain, at least in small part, the reluctance of the Euro-American communities in general and their elderly in particular to mount a campaign for support and funding comparable to those mounted by other ethnic groups.

A CLOSER LOOK AT THE IMMIGRATION COHORT

Immigrants came to the United States at different times in history and for different reasons, often for reasons that existed for that nation or region or people at that unique time. This also meant that the characteristics of the immigrants differed (Kolm, 1980). The now-elderly Poles who came to the United States to escape the onslaughts of Hitler and Stalin differed from those who came prior to World War I, even though they might now be of the same age cohort; the aging Hungarian-American freedom fighter differs in many ways from the aging Hungarian-American of the same age cohort who entered this nation as an infant.

On the whole, the more recent immigrants were better received than those who arrived during the massive immigration waves that ended in 1914, and those who are now elderly seem to have a more optimistic outlook and higher life satisfaction then the now-elderly who arrived earlier (Kolm, 1980). They led different kinds of lives before leaving their homelands, came prepared for different life-styles in this country, and have had different kinds of experiences here. While they may share language, religion, and some customs with earlier immigrants, the later immigrants also differ in many ways.

For the most part, later immigrant cohorts, including recent immigrants, were greeted by their predecessors with warmth, cordiality, and often a great deal of help in their early adjustment. They would be housed, fed, helped to get jobs, and introduced to the culture.

However, relationships between early immigrants and recent cohorts from the same ethnic community were not always completely cordial. For example, those Greeks who arrived after 1965 viewed earlier Greek immigrants as socially and intellectually inferior, while the latter group would sometimes describe the former as "arrogant, pretentious, boisterous, and overly demanding" (Saloutos, 1980, p. 437). Similarly, post-World War II immigrants from Romania and Poland were more likely to be middle-class, moderately or well educated, and qualified for professional or managerial jobs. This sometimes produced tensions for them in their contacts with earlier arrivals who entered the United States from agricultural or unskilled-work backgrounds (Bobango, 1980; Greene, 1980).

In other instances, differences between early and recent immigrants had political overtones. Thus, the Serbs who came just after World War II and those who arrived earlier were interested in political issues; those who arrived during the past 15 or so years had fewer political interests, and the ones they had were normally unrelated to World War II issues (Petrovich & Halpern, 1980). Conflicts developed between Czechs who were brought up under socialism and those reared under democratic regimes, either in Czechoslovakia or the United States (Freeze, 1980).

It is also important to point out that the situation for post-World War II immigrants in the United States was no longer the same as it had been prior to World War I or during the Depression. From the late 1940s virtually to the present, jobs were more plentiful, especially for those who arrived with some skills. There were many people of the various ethnic groups already here to make adjustment easier; many of them were established in careers and in the wider community. The ethnic hostility with which immigrants were often met in earlier times was no longer directed at European immigrants. Relatively few of either the original immigrants or the newcomers lived in poverty.

That tensions developed between immigration cohorts within the same ethnic groups should be no more surprising than the fact that tensions can develop within families or within a church congregation. The tensions seem to be based on differences in social status (the newcomers frequently had higher status), in generation (the newcomers were almost always younger), and in political and social values (the newcomers were more influenced by the recent political views of the homeland). However, it is important that discussion of the differences not draw attention from the help that each immigrant cohort has offered the other, nor from the basically cordial relationships that exist among them as individuals.

It would be a mistake to assume that all Euro-American groups followed the same immigration pattern. Thus, virtually none of the elderly Estonians or Latvians interviewed by Guttmann et al. (1979a) in the Baltimore area had arrived in this country prior to 1938. More than half of the Estonians and more than 40% of the Latvians reached the United States during the 1940s. (We need to be cautious, however, in interpreting these data since they might be specific to Guttmann's sample, but they also seem to make the point.)

Obviously, each new generation will differ from previous generations, and this is as true for Euro-American communities as for the general community. This concept can also be viewed in terms of Euro-American elderly: those who may be defined as Euro-American elderly during one decade may differ from those similarly defined a decade earlier.

Given the inevitability of change and without trying to second-guess the future, what has been happening with Euro-American group identification? A statement by the authors of an article on ethnically relevant survey research is probably applicable to Euro-Americans in general and Euro-American elderly in particular: "Perhaps the most important overall generalization on the basis of the evidence . . . is that the effect of ethnicity has tended to diminish in the public sphere—in the occupational structure, levels of educational attainment, and economic position—but not in the private sphere" (Wright, Rossi, & Juravich, 1980, p. 970). The *private sphere* refers to such factors as selection of and relationships with neighbors, neighborhoods, friends, spouses, and non-nuclear family members. This author would also like to include in the private sphere participation in some ethnic celebrations, recognition of the tie between ethnicity and religion, and a definite sense of identification of oneself as a member of the ethnic community.

It would seem that those who develop policy or plan or conduct programs that affect Euro-American elderly need to attend to these findings. Previous assumptions appear either to follow the notion that the status quo will remain forever or that Euro-American group identification will soon cease to require attention. If the authors cited above are correct, ethnicity will continue to be a signficant factor in the lives of the elderly of coming decades, but not in precisely the same form as in the past, or even the recent past.

VALUES AND THEIR SIGNIFICANCE

Those who share ethnic group membership also tend to share values. If age-cohort status and immigration-cohort status are also shared, the chances for sharing values are increased considerably.

These values are an integral part of being a member of that ethnic group. As was stated in the opening paragraph of this chapter, ethnicity is a way of life, and values that are part of the ethnic tradition are similarly part of this way of life.

These comments should not be interpreted to mean that membership in an ethnic group fully determines an individual's values. Each person is a member of numerous groups and sub-groups, and each person is also unique in his or her own right. Thus, ethnicity becomes only one of many sources of the develop-ment of values, albeit, for many people, a particularly important one. Since the elderly are more likely than their younger counter-parts to have been brought up in an ethnic community, to have lived in an ethnic neighborhood, and to have been socialized in a family setting in which ethnic values permeated everything that went on, Euro-American elderly are frequently more influenced by traditional values than the non-elderly.

Traditional Values

Early European-American immigrants frequently attempted to re-create in this country the family systems and value systems that they had experienced in their homelands. At the present time, however, these systems "are no longer transplanted social entities but have become integral to a distinctive type of pluralist society whose internal differences are more likely to be home grown than imported" (Habenstein & Mindel, 1981, p. 424). Although these authors were applying their statement to ethnic families in general and not to Euro-American situations, their words seem valid for our purposes also.

However, today's elderly Euro-Americans may be a transitional group, initially socialized to the very traditional and now living in the contemporary. Their traditional values include strong family-centered views; the family is the most important unit for identity, loyalties, and social organization. Family structure is authoritarian, headed by the father but centered around the mother; gender and age roles are carefully delineated (Habenstein & Mindel, 1981).

Religious values and church affiliation are key elements in the lives of the Euro-American elderly, as are patriotic values and a strong support for the United States. These views certainly do not exclude criticism of either church or country, but essential sup-port for both institutions appears firm. Similarly, the history of unions is very much a part of the history of the Euro-American elderly; they participated actively in unions, and their own power and influence were extended by unions (Habenstein & Mindel, 1984). These were blue-collar unions, however, and membership in recent years has diminished; white-collar unions, which tend not to have Euro-American identification, are on the rise. Therefore, it would appear to this author that identification with unions may be a diminishing factor to the Euro-American elderly of the future.

Another entrenched value of the present generation of elderly is the value of work and of developing self-help organizations in opposition to the extension of welfare and government intervention. Many Euro-American groups emphasized the importance of preparing for and getting a good job in order to avoid financial dependence on both agencies and individuals, then settling down and having a family (Habenstein & Mindel, 1981).

Ethnically derived values also emerge in other arenas. For example, responses to the educational system are often strongly affected by ethnicity. Public schools in the United States have traditionally been strongly assimilationistic, and while most ethnic group members wished to become Americans, they did not want to do so at the price of rejecting family and group values (Olneck & Lazerson, 1980). Since public schools were dominated by Protestants, those Euro-American group members who were Catholic often began their own schools, frequently focused not just on Roman Catholicism or Greek Orthodoxy, but on specific ethnic group values, customs, and history. Even textbooks were often unsatisfactory because they also tended to emphasize national unity rather than diversity of origins or cultures (Olneck & Lazerson, 1980).

For many Euro-American communities, education was a means to a good job, but not particularly important in its own right (Habenstein & Mindel, 1981). This view might reflect either their experiences with education prior to coming to the United States or their experiences after arriving. For example, Slavic immigrants sometimes viewed the public schools as promoting assimilation. Since they were likely to believe the purpose of education was for cultural continuity and maintaining ethnically acceptable values, they often did not encourage extensive education. Similarly, early immigrants from southern Italy believed that both religious and secular knowledge were available through community folklore and that formal education in the public schools would not enhance this knowledge (Olneck & Lazerson, 1980). Although these two examples are not contemporary, and members of these and other Euro-American groups are avidly pursuing education, the effects on older Europeans are sometimes still in evidence.

A similar experience can be found in attitudes and values regarding health. Many early immigrants and their children retained the health beliefs and practices of their homelands, including what has been at various times derided and lauded as folk medicine and folk healers (Chrisman & Kleinman, 1980). However, Euro-American elderly are affected in their pursuit of good health by much more than what is often termed folk medicine. The entire issue of causality, how illnesses come about and why, is influenced by ethnic values. For example, although physicians believe that colds come from viruses, many Americans assume that dampness causes colds (Chrisman & Kleinman, 1980).

Other health-related issues include perceptions of pain, how severe symptoms must be before they seek help, where they go for help, and whether they prefer a physician of their own ethnic group (Chrisman & Kleinman, 1980). Since ethnic values may also lead some people to believe that their own "evil" deeds cause their illness, and since contemporary psychology in its own way supports this, an intriguing mix of old and new becomes involved in health care and most certainly in any sort of preventive maintenance.

All of the foregoing is strongly influenced by age cohort and by immigration cohort. In a relatively few years, the Euro-American elderly will be composed almost completely of those who are American-born and reared, or those who immigrated to this country as adults in the post-World War II period. As that occurs, the values and resulting behavior and expectations of the then-elderly will change. Further, since the individuals concerned are already in this country, we can make good predictions about the nature of the changes if we are willing to undertake the necessary research. To indicate that interest in this area already exists, the 1985 Request for Proposals of the Administration on Aging emphasized the importance of learning how the non-elderly of today were preparing for the aging of tomorrow.

If there is a message in these paragraphs, it seems to this author to be that we must simultaneously attend to the needs and values of the Euro-American elderly today as we anticipate and plan for the probable needs and values of the Euro-American elderly of tomorrow.

Customs and Ceremonies

It is almost too obvious to mention, yet it can easily be ignored: sharing ethnic group membership often means sharing customs, ceremonies, and rituals. As with values, the likelihood that these will be shared is enhanced when individuals are of the same age cohort or immigration cohort. Therefore, older Slovaks may recall, either in the United States or in their homeland, wedding celebrations that lasted several days and were attended by 200 or more people, with singing, dancing, musical groups, and a variety of food. Younger people of the same ethnic group are usually aware that this is part of their tradition, but their weddings and receptions tend to last only a few hours and are attended by fewer people. However, it still tends to be important that family members are present and that traditional foods are offered (Stolarik, 1980).

Similarly, funerals, holiday celebrations, christenings, and other ceremonial events have changed in nature over the decades while still retaining great importance for older persons. One of the fears that Euro-American elderly have when they contemplate residing in a long-term care facility is that they might be isolated from the joyous occasions that are celebrated within their communities, even though these occasions differ considerably from their earlier memories.

Ethnic Pride and Ethnic Loyalties

Among the values that seem to be maintained within the ethnic community is that of strong personal pride in the ethnic group. In the research interviews conducted by Guttmann et al. (1979a), at least 90% of each of the eight ethnic groups indicated that they felt pride, usually great pride, in their ethnic group. Nearly 97% of the entire sample of 720 elderly believed that their ethnic culture should be preserved, and more than three out of four older respondents observed ethnic holidays, although responses to this question turned up substantial differences among the groups. Only 30% of the elderly Italians and 59% of the elderly Hungarians observed ethnic holidays, compared with 95% of the Estonians and 93% of the Greeks.

Guttmann et al. (1979a) subsequently developed a four-item *ethnic feeling index,* based on the interviews conducted with these Euro-American elderly. Of these eight ethnic groups, the elderly of Lithuanian origins exhibited the strongest ethnic feelings, while those of Hungarian background had the lowest scores. We do not know, of course, whether these findings are generalized beyond the Baltimore and Washington, DC, areas where the investigation was conducted, but they provide important initial data.

Other questions in the same study confirmed the strength of ethnic pride. Thus, virtually all respondents wanted the next generation to develop strong ethnic identification and to internalize the values and customs of their ethnic group. More than half preferred contact with members of their own ethnic group to contact with persons of other ethnic communities (Guttmann et al., 1979a), although this latter finding need not be interpreted as representing ethnic pride.

Matters of ethnic pride and ethnic identification may also affect reactions to long-term care facilities for the elderly. It was mentioned earlier that such facilities, especially if located some distance from the ethnic neighborhood, may serve to isolate the institutionalized older person from a major source of personal satisfaction. In addition, language problems that might have been mild or modest in earlier decades can, because of forgetting more recent learning, cause some frail elderly to lose all ability in English. Frequently, there is no one in the facility who can speak their language, and their isolation becomes still greater. Other symbols of their ethnic identification such as food, newspapers, clergy, and so forth, may also be absent. Those individuals who have spent their entire lives in an ethnic neighborhood both misunderstand persons not of their ethnic group and, not without cause, also greatly fear being misunderstood. It should, therefore, be no surprise that Guttmann et al. (1979a) found that nearly two thirds of the Euro-American elderly they interviewed preferred to have their own ethnic group members staff long-term care facilities for the elderly. Among the Latvian, Lithuanian, and Greek respondents, more than three times as many preferred ethnic staffing as indicated no preference.

The issues discussed above deserve further comment. Agencies and programs for the elderly in this country operate on the basis of not showing favoritism to any one ethnic group and of bringing together people of diverse ethnic backgrounds. Furthermore, to discriminate by providing jobs primarily to people of the ethnic group being served could arouse criticism from the general community. Thus, we have a definite preference stated by older Euro-Americans for having primary contact with their own ethnic group cohorts and for having ethnic group members to staff long-term care facilities. At the same time, at both national and local levels we have laws, policies, and values that oppose any kind of ethnic preference in giving services or jobs. To some extent, this issue will be solved informally and unofficially, but it may emerge from time to time to provide tension between service providers and Euro-American elderly service recipients or between government representatives and both providers and recipients.

Ethnic pride and ethnic loyalties are very similiar concepts, and over the years some individuals have accused members of certain ethnic groups of having divided national loyalties. As is often the case, since the elderly are more likely to be immigrants and closer to their ethnic communities, many of today's older Euro-Americans have been victims of these accusations. During World War I, for example, the German-American community was accused of, and sometimes vilified for, their presumed support of the Kaiser. During World War II Japanese Americans were incarcerated under much the same circumstances. However, after each war, when calmness and reason replaced wartime fervor, it was understood that the German Americans and Japanese Americans had been victimized by those who could not differentiate between ethnic loyalties and national loyalties.

Such loyalty to homeland culture can be exhibited without any sense of favoring a foreign government or nation to the detriment of loyalty to the United States government. Thus, some Euro-American elderly anticipate returning to their lands of origin, and they may feel more like visitors than residents in this country. The Serbians, for example, sometimes retire to Yugoslavia and live comfortably on Social Security (Petrovich & Halpern, 1980). Older Carpatho-Ruthenians, however, face a different situation when they return to their homeland. Their language is no longer spoken, and their home communities are split between Czechoslovakia and the Ukraine. Thus, in effect, they have no home*land* to which to return. This has created difficulties for many elderly who have gone back, either for a visit or to explore the possibility of remaining (Magocsi, 1980).

Sometimes, of course, older Euro-Americans find that the situation in their homeland has changed so much since they left that they cannot go home again. This may have been caused by a government, often Communist, that has altered certain values in the country to an extent that is upsetting for the returning older person. However, on other occasions, the changes have been produced by industrialization, urbanization, liberalization of religious and social views, and other factors that have led to comparable changes in the United States.

Ethnic loyalties have developed in another way that often goes unrecognized. In some instances, experiences in the United States have served to forge stronger ethnic identification than existed in the homeland. Thus, Greek immigrants, especially those for whom financial, political, or personal reasons made return to Greece impossible, sometimes became more intense in their ethnic feelings as they grew older. They realized that they would never return to their homeland and that whatever they valued that was Greek would need to be developed here (Saloutos, 1980). In a different context, Italian immigrants often arrived from parts of Italy that were in conflict with each other, but in the United States their identification as ethnic Italian Americans overrode regional loyalties, and a sense of unity formed that was unknown in Italy (Nelli, 1980).

CONCLUSION

What does membership in a Euro-American community offer? A group identification in which to take pride, a feeling of belonging, a link to the past and with one's roots, and a setting in which one feels comfortable and at home. It offers an opportunity to be where comments do not require translation, where shared meanings permit predictable responses, where life histories have unfolded over the years, and where the older person is recognized in terms of his or her life history, family, friends, accomplishments, and personal worth.

Whatever its physical setting, it "provides security of belonging, participation, cultural involvement, and personal identity; it also sustains capacity for coping with stress and provides communal support systems. . . . antidotes to excessive individualism, alienation, and anomie of modern mass culture" (President's Commission on Mental Health, 1978, p. 61).

In retirement people become more involved with community leadership (Kolm, 1980). They feel great ethnic pride and want their heritage and traditions handed down across the generations. They accept outsiders but prefer insiders. All of this is the ethnic community at its best.

What is the ethnic community at its worst? "Ethnocentrism,

withdrawal, clannishness, social rigidity, prejudice, and tendency toward intergroup conflict" (President's Commission on Mental Health, 1978, p. 62). Those elderly who are caught too tightly in the web of their ethnic community may be confronted with some obvious problems: difficulty in dealing with the general community, its institutions, and bureaucracies; problems in understanding and being understood due to limited skills in English; problems in knowing about, locating, accepting, and utilizing services provided by the general community. All of these concerns will be discussed more thoroughly in subsequent chapters.

One more point requires stating. The advantages listed for being tied to an ethnic community involve individual well-being and assume the availability of an informal network that functions within the community. When this is lacking, it is necessary that some formal network be available within the community for the Euro-American elderly. However, in many instances there is no operative formal network; thus, if the informal network is not available or does not exist, the older person is particularly at jeopardy. As Zev Harel states in his chapter in this volume, the "aged with high ethnic connectedness and limited levels of acculturation who lack an informal support system may be the most vulnerable and are likely to have the most extensive degree of unmet service needs" (p. 156).

It is possible to overestimate the influence of ethnic group membership on older persons because many other factors participate in their becoming who they are. However, we do not believe that this has occurred, and we are especially doubtful that this has occurred among Euro-American elderly. If anything, the meaning of ethnicity has been undervalued because it has not received the kind of attention that it has received among Black, Hispanic, Asian-American, and Native American ethnic communities. In many instances all Euro-American elderly are considered as White and thereby to have the same needs, concerns, values, and other qualities that are presumably found among prototypical middle-class White suburbanites. This book is part of what we hope is a growing effort to recognize and respect the meanings of ethnic group membership for older Euro-Americans.

3

The Significance of Language and Cultural Barriers for the Euro-American Elderly

Terrence G. Wiley, M.A.

A person's ethnic identification can be determined in a variety of ways. However, regardless of what criteria one uses to categorize oneself or others, language is often a key to identifying one's group membership. Moreover, it is also central to one's sense of identity.

In this chapter* we will address several questions regarding the significance of language and cultural barriers with reference to the Euro-American elderly. First we will take a brief historical look at attitudes of the English-speaking majority toward minorities' languages in the United States. Next we will explore various reasons why many elderly Euro-Americans persist in using their native languages or fail to become proficient in English. Then we will attempt to determine how serious the problem is and will survey various options that may be open to agencies providing services to elderly Euro-Americans. We will conclude by looking at projections for the future.

*The author wishes to express special thanks to Dr. Reynaldo F. Macías of the University of Southern California and Dr. Stephen B. Ross of California State University, Long Beach, for their comments and suggestions on earlier versions of this chapter.

A BRIEF HISTORICAL SKETCH OF LANGUAGE ATTITUDES IN THE UNITED STATES

In many countries around the world, language differences are considered normal, but in the United States speaking a language other than English has often been experienced by the non-English-speaker as a matter of shame rather than of pride (Simon, 1980). If persons do not speak English fluently, they are said to have a "language problem" regardless of how many other languages they may speak. To the extent that the inability to speak fluent English results in a denial of social benefits to which one is legally entitled it may be conceded that there is a language problem. However, the problem rests not only with the non-English-speaking individual but also with the language attitudes of the majority.

Language attitudes are deeply rooted. Senator Paul Simon (1980) in his popular book *The Tongue-tied American* has said: "Pride in a language is easily confused with nationalism or regionalism. Wars have been fought over attempts to impose another language on a people. . . . To suggest that we should learn a second language is somehow an insult to our nationhood, to our self-image" (pp. 62–63).

Whereas many English speakers would find it an infringement on their rights to be required to learn and speak a language other than English, both today and historically, the English-speaking majority has held a general expectation that non-English-speakers will and should acquire English and eventually cease using their native tongues (Macías, 1984b). Many even support a movement to make English the official language of the United States. (No official language was designated in the Constitution.) Language expectations have largely been tied to the popular belief that immigrants must undergo a process of Americanization as a kind of initiation that makes one suitable for life in the United States. An early expression of the idea can be found in the writings of a French settler, Hector St. John de Crevecoeur. In 1782, Crevecoeur defined an American as one "who has left behind him all his ancient prejudices and manners" (Pitt, 1976, p. 101). One of the manners which most Anglo-Americans wished to see left behind was the use of non-English languages.

By the time of the first United States census in 1790, some 49% of the population indicated that they were of English origin. However, despite the predominance of the English language and institutions, many of our early leaders, such as Jefferson and Franklin, were still suspicious of non-English-speaking immigrants. Franklin, for example, felt that German immigrants were clannish, loyal to Old World ways, and woefully ignorant of the English language (Pitt, 1976). Senator Paul Simon (1980) has noted that the word *foreign* has a negative connotation in the United States. Consequently, throughout our history the expectation that immigrants must undergo Americanization has persisted. It has even been argued that Americanization is a necessary test of loyalty for newcomers. Anglo-conformity has been seen as a kind of necessary price of admission.

Ironically, indigenous non-English-speaking people have also been subjected to the same logic even though they were not foreign. Although these groups are not the focus of this chapter, in order to better understand the historical context of language attitudes, we should recall that many non-English-speaking peoples such as American Indians speak indigenous languages. French-speaking and Spanish-speaking populations were acquired by the United States as a result of purchase, conquest, or colonial expansion, as in the cases of the Louisiana Purchase, the Mexican–American War, and the acquisitions of Hawaii and Puerto Rico (Macías, 1984b). Nor has the United States been alone in such attempts. Both Spain and Mexico have employed similar policies toward various Indian groups living in what is the southwestern United States and northern Mexico. (For an in-depth discussion of language policies toward Indians in the Southwest see Spicer, 1981.)

Ultimately, Americanization and Anglo-conformity may be considered expectations that the majority have for immigrants and other language minorities. They are intended, in large part, to promote assimilation. Cultural assimilation may be defined as "a cultural change of the individual and of the group, in contact situations, where the direction of the change is primarily from one group to the other (often as the result of an unequal status and power relationship)" (Macías, 1984a, p. 2).

In the early twentieth century suspicions regarding immigrants and non-English Euro-Americans peaked. For German-speaking Americans, the expectation of Anglo-conformity gave way to coercion. By 1910, 23% of the nearly 13 million foreign-born population (aged 10 years and older) did not speak English (Luebke, 1980). The more benign form of the assimilationists' expectation was expressed in the popular metaphor of "the melting pot." *The Melting Pot* was a popular play first staged in 1908 by an English–Jewish writer, Israel Zangwill (Banks, 1984). Zangwill's early-twentieth-century theme was similar to Crevecoeur's late-eighteenth-century theme although the cast of characters had begun to change. For Zangwill, in the United States " 'the great Alchemist melts and fuses [immigrants] with his purging flame— Celt and Latin, Slav and Teuton, Greek and Syrian' " (quoted in Petersen, Novak, & Gleason, 1982, p. 13).

Despite the play's popularity other sentiments were also being expressed in the political arena. Efforts were underway to restrict immigration. In 1907 the Dillingham Commission had argued that eastern and southern Europeans were fundamentally different from (and, by implication, inferior to) western Europeans (Banks, 1984). In the previous year an English language requirement had been added to other requirements for citizenship. Non-Englishspeakers had now joined "convicts, prostitutes, idiots, lunatics, and persons likely to be public charges" as those to be excluded (Leibowitz, 1984, p. 34). Though many argued that the purpose of English language requirements for citizenship and naturalization was to promote participation in democratic institutions as well as to better facilitate harmonious social and economic relations, Leibowitz suggests another purpose:

> Both the literacy requirement for immigration and the English literacy requirement for naturalization had at their root a racial purpose. They were reinforced by a series of other statutes imposing English language requirements as a condition for access to the American political and economic life.
>
> The immigration and naturalization requirements did not fulfill their purpose. In immigration, the national origin requirements rapidly overtook and made irrelevant the literacy requirement in immigration. The English language nationalization requirement, on the other hand, seems to be sustained by its rather soft enforcement and the need of immigrants to master English to advance their position and earnings potential. (p. 58)

Racial purity, however, was not the only motivation for language conformity since even German-Americans were severely ostracized for their persistence in speaking German. With the outbreak of World War I, superpatriots attacked the use of German not only in public education but even in churches:

> A mob spirit took over in some communities. German Americans were subjected to threats, intimidations, beatings, tar-and-featherings, flag-kissing ceremonies, and star chamber proceedings in council of defense meetings. Their homes and buildings received liberal applications of yellow paint as a symbol

of disloyalty. In Texas a German Lutheran pastor was whipped after he allegedly continued to preach in German. . . . In Nebraska a German Lutheran pastor was beaten by a mob. (Luebke, 1980, p. 9).

In recent years efforts by the English-speaking majority to control the use of non-English languages have been reflected in the efforts of local governments to pass restrictions on the use of foreign languages in advertising, in attempts to pass English-only rules for the work place, and in calls for a constitutional amendment that would make English the official language of the United States. Despite such moves, attitudes of the majority are generally more tolerant today than in the past, though Euro-Americans and other language minorities who do not speak fluent English are still likely to be characterized as being poorly adjusted.

Among those who provide services to non-English-speaking Euro-Americans and other language minorities, language services such as translation and interpretation are often seen as temporary support services—when they are provided at all. The assumption seems to be that the problem of not speaking English will eventually correct itself. Consequently, language support services are seen as unnecessary luxuries or as special privileges granted to language minorities. Rarely are such services viewed as an integral part of a service delivery system. Unfortunately, this view is both historically inaccurate and unrealistic. Even during periods of relative isolationism the United States has never completely closed its doors. In the case of indigenous peoples such as some Native Americans, more than 400 years of successive attempts to eradicate their native languages have failed. Nor would a constitutional amendment help to eradicate languages other than English. At best, attempts to legislate language use merely heighten awareness of language differences and increase tension between the majority of the people and the language minorities. Language shift toward English has been an ongoing process throughout our history, but it does not happen all at once, nor is it facilitated by being forced. Particularly for non-English-speaking elderly, little could be gained by trying to require them to use English.

WHY MANY HAVE NOT BECOME PROFICIENT IN ENGLISH

There are numerous factors that can account for some Euro-Americans and other language minorities retaining their native languages and failing to acquire fluency in English. Moreover, there are many reasons why people come to this country. Many come seeking a better life and economic opportunities. Others, such as refugees, come not so much by choice as by necessity. Others come to reunite with family members. Although most have seen the advantages of learning English, motivation, education, ability, and opportunity to learn vary from individual to individual.

The process whereby language minorities gradually cease using their native languages and assimilate into the world of the English-speaking majority is called *anglicanization* (Veltman, 1983). The opposite process is called *language loyalty;* that is, members of a group continue to retain their native language (Fishman, 1966, 1980). Among some groups it is typical that children born in the United States are fluent in their parents' native language. Language loyalty is manifested by the presence of non-English newspapers, radio and television programs, churches, schools, and social organizations, which are the traditional mechanisms by which ethnic groups maintain not only their language but also ethnic group awareness and identity.

Attempts to measure language loyalty have been based, at least in part, on analysis of U.S. census data. According to Che-Fu Lee's analysis of the 1980 census, a majority of Euro-Americans over the age of 65 speak languages other than English (see Chapter 4).

Which Groups Are Most Likely to Have Limited Proficiency in English?

In designing programs for elderly Euro-Americans, it is essential to know more than just how many elderly Euro-Americans speak other languages. They may speak their mother tongue but also have some ability to speak English. In Che-Fu Lee's profile of elderly European immigrants in New York City, for example, among Italian men aged 65 to 69 years he found that nearly 80% speak Italian while approximately 34% reported that they do not speak English well. Since their English proficiency is based on self-assessment, it is difficult to determine what "not speaking English well" means in terms of ability to function and gain access to needed services. This is because the census question is based on oral ability in English and does not address whether one is functionally literate in English. It is significant that nearly 75% of Italian men 65 to 69 reported less than high school education because the evidence is strong that the majority of those who are functionally illiterate in the United States are found among those who have failed to graduate from high school. Literacy researchers argue that literacy is simultaneously a statement about reading abilities and an articulation of far broader cultural and social content (Hunter & Harman, 1985). In other words, for full participation in society and for full access to services one would need to be both literate and knowledgeable of its social and cultural institutions and services.

Consequently, concern over language ability should not be merely related to oral proficiency but should also be extended to functional literacy. To the extent that many elderly Euro-Americans are not functionally literate in English, special consideration may be needed to ensure access to services and programs.

When we attempt to profile those Euro-Americans who are most likely to be either unable to speak English or to have limited fluency in English, the following picture emerges: Typically, we find elderly Greek, Polish, and Italian immigrants. For this group, low competence was most often reported among the more recent immigrants (Veltman, 1983).

Caution should be used in limiting concern only to these groups because individuals from other groups may also have limited English fluency. In fact, in some cases it is possible to find elderly Euro-Americans who have lived in the United States for most of their adult lives without becoming fluent in English. To many people this may seem strange because it is obvious that there are both social and economic advantages to becoming fluent in English. But despite the advantages of learning English, there are many reasons why many Euro-American elderly maintain loyalty to their native languages.

Language and One's Sense of Cultural Identity

One major reason for language loyalty is the relationship between one's language and one's sense of cultural identity. Frank (1980), in a three-generational study, found that after 50 years' residence in the United States, the Orthodox Jewish grandmother still prefers speaking, reading, and writing Yiddish even though her ability is adequate in English. Similarly, Bengtson (1979) found that the need to retain ethnic identity had become a virtual career among elderly Jewish and Polish Americans. Retaining the native language is not only important for one's personal sense of identity, it is also significant as a means of promoting group survival and for transmitting cultural values from one generation to the next (Mostwin, 1979). Here, it is important to recognize that one is exercising an individual choice in language use, and that such choices are often not without conflict. Immigrants are often caught between choosing to adjust to their new society and choosing to maintain relationships within their own groups, as Saville-Troike (1978) indicates:

> Those who value their own group membership and don't wish to acculturate to the dominant group may be treated as not "well adjusted" to our society. Those who reject their group and wish to change may be viewed as "traitors" to family and old friends. Those who wish to belong to more than one group may be mistrusted by both, and seen as "spies." (p. 11)

Ethnic Communities and Language Maintenance

For some elderly Euro-Americans it has been preferable to live within the United States for many years with little proficiency in English. For example, among Greeks it is not uncommon to find individuals who immigrated during the 1940s and 1950s but are scarcely fluent in English. Living within Greek-American communities it has been possible to conduct most of one's business in Greek. Religious services are conducted in Greek; schools run by Greek Orthodox churches in Greek (generally on weekends) supplement public instruction and provide a means for transmitting language and cultural values to the second and even third generations. For non-English-speaking adults, contacts with the English-speaking world are mediated by bilingual Greek-American children who have found themselves in the role of translators at such places as banks and hospitals (McMullin, 1985). For both the adults and their children, communication with the English-speaking world is frequently less than ideal, and again we may well ask why such individuals have not made a greater effort to learn English.

The Age Factor in Second Language Learning

In attempting to determine which factors facilitate or hinder language learning among elderly Euro-Americans and other aged language minorities, we should not overlook the age factor in predicting the likelihood of an individual's success in acquiring a second language. Unfortunately, a recent survey of the literature related to age and second language learning (Hatch, 1983) reveals that little research has focused on elderly learners. However, one study cited by Hatch (the *Heidelberger Forschungsprojekt,* 1978) indicates that an immigrant's age on arrival in his/her new country correlates with his/her success in learning the language. As we might expect, the older the immigrant is upon arrival, the lower his/her second language proficiency is when measured by standardized tests.

In addition to the problem of difficulties in language learning that may be attributed to advanced age, the problem of language loss is sometimes attributable to various forms of dementia. As dementia progresses, it is not unusual for an elderly person who speaks English as a second language to lose the use of English, even though that language was mastered many years earlier. Richard Kalish (personal communication, August 1985) has pointed out to the author that such cognitive regression may result in greater isolation and stress for Euro-Americans and other language minorities because they may have greater difficulty in communicating with their English-speaking adult children or with their English-speaking peers (as in the case of those who are institutionalized in long-term care facilities).

Physical Impairments and Language Loss

Language loss is also common in aphasia that results from injury to the brain. Although most bilingual people seem to experience parallel loss of facility in the languages they speak, sometimes they experience unequal loss:

> [S]ome recover one language and, as the second begins to come back, lose the first one again; some retain/recover parts of each of the languages—perhaps reading and writing skills in one language, comprehension in the same language, but production in the other. (Hatch, 1983, p. 215)

Motivation to Learn a Second Language

Motivation is obviously another key to predicting an individual's likelihood of success in acquiring a second language. Taylor (1974) has argued that affective factors may be even more important than other factors such as age. He maintains that the primary ingredient for successful second language learning among adults is a positive attitude toward the new language and culture. Conversely, the lack of positive attitudes toward the ability to speak more than one language may explain why more English-speaking Americans do not speak another language (Hill, 1970).

Given the economic and social advantages of being fluent in English, most immigrants would seem favorably predisposed to learn the language. Unfortunately, an individual who lacks fluency can experience frustration in trying to use English and therefore avoid using the language. Why is this so?

Perdue (1984) explains that when speakers of the dominant language (in this case English) have stereotyped views of ethnic minorities, lack of fluency by language minorities tends to reinforce the majority's prejudices. Many among the English-speaking majority seem to have little patience for foreign accents and so-called "broken English." Not only is one expected to use English, but one is expected to be fluent in English. When an individual is in the process of learning a second language, lack of proficiency is normal. However, many native speakers of English misinterpret errors in grammar as signs of low intelligence, poor education, or both. Consequently, for many, and especially for elderly adults, the process of learning and using English has been a difficult and frustrating experience.

Erickson (1975) and Perdue (1984) have analyzed the social context in which communication between language minorities and members of the dominant language and culture occur. When a language minority seeks social services such as welfare or health care to which he/she is legally entitled, the individual providing services (such as an eligibility worker or nurse) is often a member of the majority culture and a native speaker of English.

Consider the following familiar circumstance in which an elderly immigrant or language minority person must undergo screening from an eligibility worker before he/she can receive needed services. Typically, the eligibility worker is primarily concerned with the job, with routine, and with the number of clients that must be served. When there are dealings with language minorities, it is related only to the job. Consequently, the eligibility worker sees them only in the context of wanting something. They seem to be motivated only by their self-interest. The worker interprets their lack of competence in English as proof of the suspicion that they are ignorant or stupid. If only they could speak English, the worker could do the job more easily. From the perspective of the language minorities who seek services from the eligibility worker, he/she seems impatient, demanding, or uninterested in their personal problems. When they try to express themselves through their limited English, they feel frustration and sometimes even shame. (This hypothetical situation is extrapolated from Perdue's [1984] discussion of encounters between non-native speakers and gatekeepers, that is, those individuals who control access to services. Perdue provides many other unusual examples of problems that non-native speakers encounter when attempting to learn and use a foreign language.)

Unfortunately, negative attitudes such as these can reduce the motivation of language minorities to use and improve their English. For many elderly Euro-Americans, it may have become a matter of habit to avoid such encounters whenever possible, even when doing so has meant denying oneself needed services.

HOW SERIOUS IS THE PROBLEM?

Some may argue that negative encounters such as the one described above are unfortunate but unavoidable. If one does not speak English well in a predominantly English-speaking society, one should expect to have difficulties in communicating one's basic needs and wants.

Although there is cold but pragmatic logic to this argument, it fails to address the breadth of the problem and seeks to place responsibility solely on the non-English-speaker. It fails to deal with the built-in potential for bias that exists when a dominant group controls access to needed services. Erickson (1975) has suggested that one of the best ways to avoid ethnic bias in service provision is to ensure that members of an ethnic group are served by members of the same group. Kutzik (1979) notes that, historically, ethnic self-help or mutual-assistance organizations were formed for exactly this purpose.

To what extent are elderly Euro-Americans and other elderly language minorities really failing to receive needed services because of language and cultural differences? Much more research on the significance of language and cultural barriers for the aged appears to be needed, and the findings of several researchers indicate that the problem is prevalent. Peralta and Horikawa (1978) in a study of elderly Asian-Americans, for example, found

that well over 50% of the aged surveyed cited language barriers
and the absence of bicultural personnel as reasons for not receiving services. A similar study of eight elderly Euro-American groups
led Guttmann et al. (1979a) to speculate that language differences
may be a major barrier to gaining access to services, and that many
aged Euro-Americans avoid using government-offered services because of the social stigma attached to the use of non-English
languages.

WHAT OPTIONS EXIST FOR SERVICE PROVIDERS?

As we have seen, there are many reasons why elderly Euro-
Americans and other language minorities continue to speak languages other than English. For some it may be a matter of personal
choice to maintain ties with their communities, or it may be a
means for transmitting cultural values to the next generation. It
may also be because they have sought to avoid difficult and un-
comfortable situations in which using English seems too frustrating or embarrassing, or it may not be a matter of choice. It may be
a result of too few opportunities or even the result of maladies
sometimes associated with aging.

To the extent that language and cultural differences between
the community and the service provider result in an underutilization of services or a de facto denial of services, those who make
policy and those who provide services to ethnic communities
need to be more responsive to those communities. As Kutzik
(1979) has so aptly stated:

> [A] major objective of planners and providers of services to the aged should be
> to bring ethnicity and organization together to recreate at a higher level the
> natural ethnic organizational network that helped most of the aged throughout
> most of American history. A corollary objective should be to bring a sophisti-
> cated understanding of ethnicity into the policies of the "nonethnic" organiza-
> tional network of "nonsectarian" and "integrated" agencies so they can more
> adequately serve their ethnically diverse clientele. (p. 63)

Linguistic access should be a major objective of service providers. The presence of non-English-speaking people and of functional illiterates in English are facts of life in an ethnically and socially
diverse society such as ours. Consequently, to the extent that
equal opportunity of access to services is seen as a basic right of

clients and goal of service providers, alternative models should be sought.

Assessing Client Needs and Program Goals Together with the Community

To determine what type of model should be used will depend on the characteristics of the groups served, the nature of services provided, and the resources available. The first step should involve a needs assessment. Needs of recently arrived immigrants will vary from those of long-term residents. In designing access models it is important to design programs not only *for* the elderly but *with* the elderly and representatives of their ethnic communities.

Utilizing Bilingual/Bicultural Personnel

When programs provide services to large numbers of language minorities, it is essential to use bilingual and bicultural personnel. The successful use of bilingual/bicultural paraprofessionals has been previously demonstrated. In San Francisco, for example, health services have been provided to elderly Chinese Americans by using paraprofessional outreach workers to provide services to homebound non-English-speaking clients (U.S. Health Services Administration, 1973).

Providing Cross-Cultural Staff Training

In addition to using bilingual personnel, the English-speaking staff may also need training in cultural awareness and sensitivity geared specifically to the target population. English-speaking staff may also need training in how to best utilize translators because interpreters are sometimes treated more like "go-fors" than like paraprofessionals.

Recruiting Bilingual Professional Staff

Hiring interpreters is sometimes seen as an extra staff expenditure. For agencies with limited resources it may prove more realistic and beneficial to recruit bilingual professional staff over the long term rather than to hire extra paraprofessional teams.

Increasing Community Resources through Interagency Arrangements

For agencies with limited resources, interagency arrangements may facilitate a communitywide response. If possible, one agency may be able to coordinate translation and interpretation for other agencies within the community. In Long Beach such an arrangement worked successfully where one community-based organization provided translation for all local hospitals and homes for the elderly.

In the absence of a coordinating agency, local forums can be organized in which information and resource sharing are facilitated by means of informal interagency agreements. Ethnic mutual-assistance associations can sometimes assist with interpretation on a limited, voluntary basis. Care should be exercised, however, not to exploit help offered on a voluntary basis when other resources can be found. Since language access is not a temporary problem, it should not be treated as such.

Teaching English to the Elderly

Many elderly may not be able to nor desire to study English. However, for those elderly who do, much more could be done in the area of adult education. Nationwide, 68% of all adult students are enrolled in English-as-a-second-language programs (Hunter & Harman, 1985). Unfortunately, many programs do not focus on the special needs of elderly learners. Representatives of adult programs should be invited to community forums that deal with the needs of language minorities. Where the demand exists, special courses should be designed specifically to meet the needs of the elderly.

When curriculum is designed for elderly learners, an attempt should be made to identify and address the specific types of communicative needs of the learner. Emphasis should be placed on functional communication and social interaction. Lessons can be designed around meeting various social needs. They should be designed to include needed information about available programs and services for the elderly. Specific lessons can focus on solving social interaction problems in which elderly students are taught to make appointments with doctors or service agencies, learn to call for emergency services in English, and so forth.

For successful and relevant English instruction there is a need for more interagency communication and cooperation to identify needs and goals of instruction.

CONCLUSION

In recent years, increasing recognition has been given to the notion of cultural pluralism. Cultural pluralism, as opposed to notions of assimilation such as Americanization and Anglo-conformity, implies "conditions that produce sustained ethnic differentiation and continued heterogeneity" (Abramson, 1980, p. 150).

Recent language projections indicate that by the year 2000 we will witness an increase in the number of individuals over the age of 55 who speak languages other than English. For example, according to Oxford (1980), the Italian-speaking population over the age of 55 is projected to increase by more than 400,000 (from 1.2 million in 1976 to over 1.6 million by the year 2000). Similarly, the Polish-speaking population over the age of 55 is expected to increase by more than 200,000 (from 0.8 million in 1976 to over 1 million by the year 2000).

If we are to do more than pay mere lip service to cultural pluralism, we as a nation and we as service providers need to accept diversity as representative of the human condition rather than seeing it as a deviation. Beyond the issues of utilization of services is the issue of whether or not linguistic access should be a fundamental human right. Although the United Nations has taken the position that one should have a fundamental right to speak one's native language, many in the United States today would support a constitutional amendment making English the official language. For a fuller discussion of the language rights issue see Macías (1979) and Kloss (1971, 1977). Language choice may eventually come to be viewed as a basic human right.

Anyone who has traveled to a foreign country knows how difficult life can become when he/she does not speak the language of the majority. Normal communication can be frustrating, and problem situations can become a matter of life and death in an emergency situation. Yet some have bluntly argued that we should not coddle those who do not speak English by providing translation and interpretation or cross-cultural assistance, even when failure to provide such services may in many cases be tantamount to a denial of services. The language problem can be solved, in large part, by recognizing that language diversity has always been a fact of life. Such diversity does not threaten the dominance of English. It has predominated since early in our history, and despite occasional paranoiac fears to the contrary, its dominance continues unchallenged. Language and cultural diversity have always coexisted with that dominance and will continue to do so. Once this is acknowledged, we can better develop a more realistic and egalitarian response to what Joshua Fishman (1981) has termed the *little languages.* With him let us agree that:

> A world made safe for little languages, through which people feel deeply and think creatively, would be a better, more human, more accepting and more innovative world for one and for all.
>
> Languages must be shared as a common good, they must be saved, loved, treasured. National policy toward this end finally lifts languages off of the ethnicity versus anti-ethnicity treadmill and sets them into a new universal orbit in which uniqueness serves not itself but the general good. (p. 524)

Senator Simon (1980) has written: "Despite our rich ethnic mix, and despite the fact that we are the fourth largest Spanish-speaking nation in the world, we remain ignorant of languages and cultures other than our own" (p. 72). To better meet the needs of all the aged, we must promote policies that meet the needs of the present and anticipate those of the future. To do this we must improve our awareness and understanding of the diversity of cultures and languages in our country. We must promote better English educational programs for the elderly, and we must also acknowledge and promote the resources of bilingual individuals to guarantee linguistic access.

4

A Demographic Profile of Older Euro-Americans

Che-Fu Lee, Ph.D.

In a pluralistic society such as the United States, policies and programs need to be developed so that the diversity of the population is taken into consideration. To accomplish this an early step—perhaps the first step—is to obtain a clear picture of the characteristics of the members of the society. This requires having access to demographic data that is both accurate and sufficiently comprehensive to offer the needed information. To permit effective planning, such data need to describe both those characteristics that are modal for the entire population and those that pertain to limited segments of the population. For example, in serving the needs of the Polish community of Philadelphia, we would need to know both that most adult women are married and that a certain proportion of adult women are never-married, divorced, or widowed; or that most families are living well above the poverty line but that some are below the poverty line, at, or just above the line. Of course, we need to know the number and percentages in each category.

Acknowledgment is gratefully expressed to Arthur Cresce, Betsy Corcoran, and Charles Longino for acquisition of the census data; to Sharon Ardison and Karen Stevens for tabular and graphic data preparations; to Christopher Hayes and Theodora Ooms for reading and commenting on an earlier draft; and to James P. O'Connor for supporting this research, in part with university research funds. Although this chapter has been extensively revised by Richard Kalish for purposes of stylistic consistency, the basic content has not been changed from the original. Therefore, the opinions and shortcomings contained herein remain solely those of the author. For a more complete and academic statement on this issue, contact Dr. Che-Fu Lee, The Catholic University of America, Washington, DC 20064.

Because this kind of information has been available for minority groups such as Blacks, Hispanics, Asian Americans, and Native Americans, their advocates have been able to establish the needs of those individuals and to press for policies and programs to respond to those needs. The living conditions of the Euro-Americans, more particularly the Euro-American elderly, are less well known and have not been studied in detail. This lack of information weakens the case for advocacy and reduces the effectiveness of planning.

As discussed elsewhere in this volume, the terms *ethnic* and *elderly* both involve a wide range of individual interpretive meanings. In 1980 the Bureau of the Census for the first time attempted to address the subjective aspect of ethnic identification by asking respondents about their ancestry. The results showed that more than 80% identified with one, and sometimes more, ancestry groups of foreign origin (U.S. Bureau of the Census, 1983). These findings are, in themselves, interesting and undoubtedly indicative as signs of contemporary American pluralism. However, it becomes difficult to be certain as to what particular factor or factors led any given respondent to present the answer he/she gave. One's perceptions of one's own ethnicity are based on such objective factors as culture of origin, language, region, and religion, and on such subjective factors as personal orientation and preference. Thus, the basis for Person A's decision to consider himself/herself Ukrainian or Scottish may differ considerably from the same decision of Person B.

The basic definition of ethnic for this volume is broad and encompassing; it emphasizes identification and preference more than place of birth. However, for purposes of this demographic analysis we have selected a more restricted definition, that of being a first-generation immigrant and so identifying oneself. Further restricting our analysis is the fact that the individuals included must be age 65 or over and that they have provided the census taker with that information.

We selected the chronological definition of age because any other definition makes the use of census data impossible. We selected age 65 as the boundary to accord with the most familiar usage, and this is followed elsewhere in this book as much as possible. To use only the self-identification described above would, we believe, dilute the meaning of ethnicity for our purposes because the vast majority of the population applied it to themselves. Therefore, our decision to use only first-generation immigrants was made because these individuals are closest to their ethnic origins, and the numbers in most categories are adequate for this study.

BACKGROUND

Euro-American immigrants are currently overrepresented among the age categories of old (65 to 74 years) and old-old (75 years and over). (The initial categories described by Neugarten in 1974 were young-old and old-old, but her younger group began at age 55, and ours begins at 65.) This has occurred because the flow of immigrants from Europe has declined since the early decades of this century. Most immigration of the past two decades has come from Latin American and Asian nations. Of the 36 million Euro-American immigrants recorded by the annual reports of the Immigration and Naturalization Service from 1820 to 1977, only about 3 million entered the United States after 1950 (Gelfand, 1982).

Future projections for the population of the United States as a whole indicate that the old-old, those over age 75, constitute the most rapidly growing age group, with somewhat slower increases for those between 65 and 75. This expectation has already been realized for some years by the immigrant populations from Europe (U.S. Congress, House Select Committee, 1984). Thus, using our definition, older Euro-Americans are not only overrepresented among the elderly in general but also among Euro-Americans in general.

Previous studies of older Euro-Americans have been based on data collected in very limited geographical locations or through ethnographic reports. From such reports, this population might be summarized as follows:

Due to their immigration history the Euro-American populations are old and overrepresented by widowed or unmarried women. The great majority of these Euro-American elderly are living in single-person households and depend on informal social support networks for many of their needs. Although they are underrepresented among those living in poverty, their utilization of public services is still lower than expected, even when considering the relatively small proportion living in poverty. It is not known to what extent this limited utilization arises from language and cultural barriers that inhibit their search for services, as opposed to barriers imposed by service providers, but it may be assumed that both factors are involved (Guttmann et al., 1979a; Center for the Study of Pre-Retirement and Aging, 1979; White House Conference on Aging, 1981).

THE PRESENT STUDY

To provide a demographic base for this book and for the 1985 National Conference on Euro-American Elderly that led to this book, the author has examined existing census data to develop population statistics on various Euro-American ethnic communities. This will offer a way to determine the extent to which the preceding paragraph accurately describes these populations and, more important, it will provide an initial demographic analysis that can serve those who develop policies and programs for this segment of the older American population.

An initial caution: census data, like all data, are subject to a variety of possibilities of error. For example, sampling errors can occur, especially when the size of the population is small. Also, there is always the possibility that first-generation immigrants belonging to one ethnic group might be more likely to indicate their membership in that group than would members of some other first-generation immigrant group. Third, there is the possibility of some kind of systematic bias in the way certain questions are answered. For example, the old-old may distort their year of arrival in the United States more frequently than the young-old, or members of one ethnic group may exaggerate their years of formal education more than members of another group. It is obvious that there is no way to know the extent to which any of these errors may occur, and we intend to accept the data at face value, while recognizing the possibility of error.

Another limitation of these data is that they are based on country of origin rather than ethnicity. For example, the statistics on Russians will include Byelorussians, Jews, Ukrainians, and Armenians, which are each distinct ethnic groups but without representation in the data.

Sources of Data

The data come from two major sources, both derived from the returns of those individuals who filled out the long forms of the 1980 census (about 19% of all persons responding to the census).

The first of these sources was the Center for International

Research and Population, a division of the U.S. Bureau of the Census. In response to requests from international organizations, this division produced a number of special tabulations for the foreign-born population of the United States. These covered 163 different countries of birth and included data on age, gender, citizenship, marital status, labor force participation and work status, use of a language other than English, ability to speak English, and various other factors.

For this analysis we obtained data for 11 Euro-American immigrant groups having a population of 100,000 or more and coming from eastern, western, and southern European nations. Unfortunately, some of the data we desired were simply not available, such as a division into two populations of those over age 65. Therefore, this needs to be considered as an initial venture and not a definitive statement. Nonetheless, it is, to our knowledge, the first venture of its kind.

The second source of information is also based on data gathered by the U.S. census in 1980. This time we selected the microdata of five central city areas of the New York Standard Metropolitan Statistical Area. The choice was made because a large number of Euro-American immigrants, who represent a large number of countries of origin, now live in these areas. In this instance, we obtained basic data on 10 countries of origin, with more complete data for 7. Each country of origin selected met three criteria: the population was European-born; it included a large proportion of people 65 years of age and over; and there was a high proportion of people using a language other than English at home. All seven countries for which complete data were provided are in eastern or southern Europe.

The determination of which countries of birth to include was based on the apparent relevance of the immigrant population to the purposes of the conference. Therefore, some countries were eliminated because they were not represented by many immigrants; others were dropped because the barriers to service for their immigrant populations appeared minimal.

Demographic Data: The National Sample

In 1980 the population of the United States stood at 227 million persons. Of the 14 million foreign-born, 4.7 million claimed European countries of birth (News release, U.S. Bureau of the Census, October 7, 1984). Some other statistics:

- Of the 4.7 million European immigrants, 65% had entered the United States prior to 1960.
- Of those Euro-Americans who were older, more than half entered the United States before 1950.
- Of all European immigrants over the age of 5 years, 60% spoke languages other than English in their homes.
- While 11% of the entire population of the United States was over 65 years of age, 37% of Euro-American immigrants were in this age group.
- Euro-American immigrants constitute 2% of the entire U.S. population, but elderly Euro-American immigrants constitute 6% of the elderly U.S. population.
- Among elderly Euro-Americans, women outnumber men 100 to 78; the ratio for the entire elderly population is about 3 to 2.

Table 4.1 provides data on Euro-American immigrants in general. The data clearly indicate that the proportion of immigrants over the age of 65 is substantially higher than for the general population, and that this is true for every country of birth except Iceland. In several instances, more than half of the immigrants from a particular country are over age 65. Table 4.2 shows the relationship between age distribution and time of immigration. (At this point we wish to repeat a caution stated earlier: not all immigrants are members of the indicated ethnic group, and not all members of ethnic communities are immigrants. This issue has been discussed at length in Chapter 2.)

For the balance of this analysis we shall limit ourselves to the following 11 countries of birth: Austria, Czechoslovakia, France, Germany, Greece, Hungary, Italy, Netherlands, Poland, Portugal, and Yugoslavia. These are countries of birth for approximately 70% of all Euro-American immigrants and are probably the countries of origin for an equally high percentage of all Euro-ethnic people. The number of older immigrants from these nations is 1.2 million. We will also limit the analysis to those immigrants who are over 65 and who entered the United States prior to 1960.

Figure 4.1 displays clearly the overrepresentation of both elderly men and elderly women among the selected Euro-American immigrant groups. (There is, of course, a selection bias because, by limiting ourselves to persons who immigrated prior to 1960, we assured an overrepresentation of older persons.) For virtually every country of birth, in keeping with the general U.S. population,

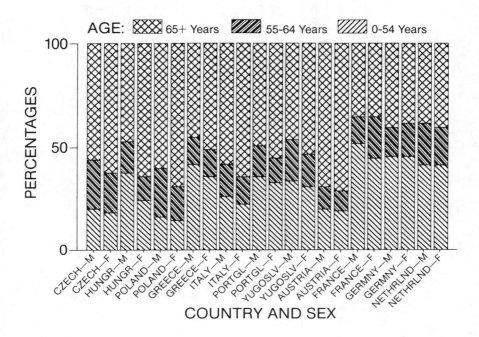

FIGURE 4.1 Age by Sex and Country—Before 1960.

the proportion of women who are elderly exceeds that of men. The reasons this is not the case for German-born or French-born immigrants are unknown, but three possibilities exist: a larger number of men immigrated initially; men have a longer life expectancy (this alternative is dubious); or younger women immigrated to this country.

The marital status of these older immigrants is shown in Figure 4.2. It will be readily noted that the differences in marital status across ethnic groups is slight, but the differences between men and women are considerable and consistent, once again paralleling the general population trends. Approximately two thirds of the older men are married in comparison to less than one third of the women. Conversely, the proportion of women who are widowed, divorced, or separated is more than twice the proportion for men. Since relatively few of these men or women are currently divorced or separated, it can only be assumed that for the older Euro-Americans as for Americans in general, the proportion of

TABLE 4.1 Euro-American Immigrant Population and Selected Characteristics, U.S. Census, 1980

Area	Total	Males per 100 females	% Immigrated 1959 or earlier	% Under 15 years	% 65 years and over	% Persons 5 years and over in households that speak non-English language
Europe	4,743,333	78.1	65.2	3.5	37.1	60.4
Eastern Europe	859,843	81.8	76.2	1.0	48.9	74.4
Bulgaria	8463	135.2	47.4	2.1	31.1	78.4
*Czechoslovakia	112,707	73.2	77.4	1.0	48.4	71.2
Estonia	12,169	77.1	87.6	1.0	42.3	79.5
*Hungary	144,368	87.3	81.0	0.7	48.0	72.1
Latvia	34,349	80.3	93.2	0.3	46.2	77.7
Lithuania	48,194	77.0	92.6	0.3	60.5	74.9
*Poland	418,128	81.2	74.5	0.9	51.1	75.8
Romania	66,994	93.7	56.0	3.4	38.1	74.5
Northern Europe	1,083,949	65.6	66.0	3.9	37.8	15.1
Denmark	42,732	95.9	72.6	2.0	47.2	51.2
Finland	29,172	56.0	69.9	2.4	50.9	72.9
Iceland	4156	59.7	41.4	13.4	9.4	57.4
Ireland	197,817	58.5	78.1	1.1	47.1	6.8
Norway	63,368	89.7	82.2	1.6	56.3	53.7
Sweden	77,157	83.6	80.5	2.0	63.4	50.7

United Kingdom	669,149	62.8	58.8	5.3	29.3	5.1
Channel Islands	704	67.6	53.8	15.2	27.3	6.6
England	442,499	61.3	56.1	6.2	26.8	5.4
Isle of Man	411	42.2	54.7	5.1	39.7	3.2
Northern Ireland	19,831	66.2	65.0	3.2	31.4	3.1
Scotland	142,001	62.6	72.2	2.3	42.2	3.0
Wales	13,528	63.7	71.0	2.1	39.9	10.5
Southern Europe	1,503,003	99.6	55.0	4.1	34.5	85.4
Albania	7381	141.4	66.4	1.2	43.9	85.9
Andorra	1201	82.5	43.0	9.2	30.1	84.6
Gibraltar	1608	60.3	44.6	9.5	24.9	68.6
*Greece	210,998	114.7	40.3	4.3	21.7	92.6
*Italy	831,922	95.6	69.8	2.1	44.5	81.4
Malta	10,182	124.7	64.1	3.4	17.2	70.2
*Portugal	211,614	100.7	21.0	10.1	14.8	94.2
San Marino	1020	130.8	48.2	9.5	17.6	84.9
Spain	73,735	99.1	30.6	8.2	29.3	86.9
*Yugoslavia	152,967	99.1	52.5	4.0	28.0	85.1
Western Europe	1,290,336	65.6	69.1	4.1	31.5	59.0
*Austria	145,607	63.4	87.9	0.9	62.7	57.2
Belgium	36,487	68.9	70.2	3.9	34.5	59.8
*France	120,215	59.2	55.0	4.7	20.4	67.9
*Germany	849,384	62.6	68.8	4.7	27.9	57.7
Luxemburg	3125	62.8	63.4	3.9	33.1	50.1
Monaco	1050	57.9	45.1	9.7	19.5	71.1
*Netherlands	103,136	96.8	66.1	2.3	27.2	59.9
Switzerland	42,804	91.7	62.4	4.6	36.3	65.9
Soviet Union	406,022	80.5	70.4	5.7	57.8	64.5

*Countries selected for further analysis in the following 2 tables.

TABLE 4.2 Number and Age Distribution by Sex and Time of Immigration for 11 Euro-American Immigrant Groups of 100,000 or more, U.S. Census, 1980

Country	Sex	Year of Immigration							
		1959 or earlier				1960–80			
		Number	% 54 & under	% 55–64	% 65+	Number	% 54 & under	% 55–64	% 65+
Czechoslovakia	M	35,215	20.2	23.6	56.1	12,412	81.8	12.0	6.2
	F	52,058	17.6	19.6	63.3	13,022	81.0	10.9	8.1
Hungary	M	53,529	38.4	14.8	46.8	13,763	79.0	10.2	10.8
	F	63,364	23.8	12.3	64.0	13,712	70.9	12.5	16.6
Poland	M	137,493	16.0	24.0	60.0	49,921	78.0	13.0	9.0
	F	174,195	14.0	17.0	69.0	56,519	78.0	12.0	10.0
Greece	M	43,687	41.6	13.8	44.7	69,021	91.5	5.7	2.8
	F	41,369	35.7	13.0	51.3	56,920	88.9	5.7	5.4
Italy	M	273,776	26.0	16.0	58.0	132,794	87.0	8.0	5.0
	F	306,686	22.0	14.0	64.0	118,666	84.0	9.0	7.0

Portugal	M	21,720	36.0	15.0	49.0	84,479	89.0	7.0	4.0
	F	22,651	33.0	12.0	55.0	82,764	87.0	8.0	5.0
Yugoslavia	M	38,107	34.3	19.7	46.0	38,031	91.2	6.1	2.7
	F	42,138	31.1	15.6	53.3	34,685	87.8	6.8	5.4
Austria	M	48,873	21.0	11.0	69.0	7,603	87.0	6.0	7.0
	F	79,180	19.0	10.0	71.0	9,951	83.0	6.0	11.0
France	M	22,127	51.8	13.3	34.9	22,575	95.3	3.0	1.8
	F	44,023	45.6	19.7	34.7	31,490	92.5	3.9	3.5
Germany	M	228,128	46.0	14.0	40.0	93,120	94.0	3.0	3.0
	F	345,865	46.0	16.0	38.0	167,999	94.0	3.0	3.0
Netherlands	M	34,172	42.5	19.1	38.4	16,553	87.4	9.0	3.6
	F	33,984	42.2	17.6	40.2	18,427	90.0	6.2	3.9

women who are widowed far exceeds the proportion of men.
These gender differences in marital status for older European
immigrants stem from a combination of three factors: women
outlive men, women marry men older than themselves, and
women are less likely to remarry after either widowhood or divorce than men.

Another noteworthy statistic indicated in Figure 4.2 is that few
older men or women are never-married. This figure is lower than
5% for the European immigrants, the same as for the elderly
population as a whole. This high probability of marrying, very
much in contrast with the contemporary trend among younger
persons in the general population, reflects values held by the
various cultures represented by these groups.

Figure 4.3 shows that first-generation Euro-American elderly
received little formal education: Just over 10% of the southern
European immigrants had completed high school; and even for the
better educated western Europeans, the proportion of high school

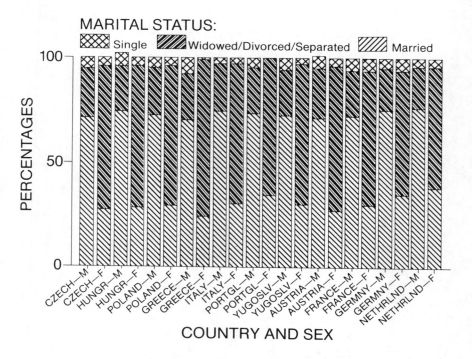

FIGURE 4.2 Marital Status by Sex and Country—65+ Years.

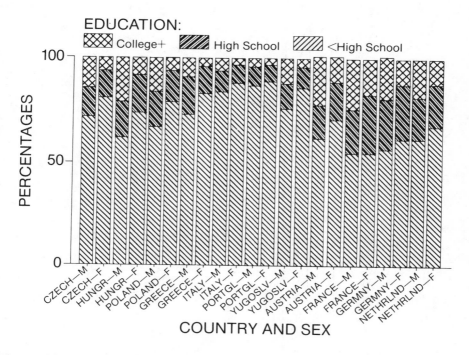

FIGURE 4.3 Education by Sex and Country—65+ Years.

graduates remained under 50%. Regardless of the country of birth, men received more formal education than women.

Table 4.3 presents a picture of labor force participation for three age stages: 55 to 59, 60 to 64, and 65+ for both male and female Euro-American immigrant groups. Consistent with their lower level of formal education, the immigrants from Greece, Italy, and Portugal have a lower level of labor force participation below age 65. The exception to this is women from the Netherlands, who have a lower level of participation than women from all other countries at each of the pre-65 categories. One explanation for the low level of labor force participation among Dutch women is that the combination of adequate-to-high incomes and traditional values permitted them to remain at home and outside the labor force. This is, of course, merely speculation.

Explaining the differences between Greece, Italy, Portugal, and the remaining countries of birth also requires speculation. The possibility arises that those with better education also had higher

TABLE 4.3 Labor Force Participation of Immigrants before 1960 by Sex for Ages 55–59, 60–64, and 65+, U.S. Census, 1980

Country	Sex	55–59 years			60–64 years			65+		
		Number	% in LF	% not	Number	% in LF	% not	Number	% in LF	% not
Czechoslovakia	M	5,449	90	10	2,875	74	26	19,762	14	86
	F	6,262	52	48	3,660	39	61	32,952	5	95
Hungary	M	4,733	90	10	3,173	75	25	25,057	18	82
	F	4,304	54	46	3,472	38	62	40,532	5	95
Poland	M	18,226	89	11	14,535	71	29	83,360	20	80
	F	18,074	51	49	11,506	34	66	120,589	6	94
Greece	M	3,028	85	15	2,980	66	34	19,525	16	84
	F	2,868	43	27	2,504	32	68	21,235	5	95
Italy	M	25,174	84	16	17,732	64	36	159,402	12	88
	F	23,982	47	53	18,087	34	66	195,730	4	96

Portugal	M	1,370	85	15	1,888	58	42	10,740	11	89
	F	1,288	51	49	1,382	34	66	12,578	4	96
Yugoslavia	M	4,513	87	13	2,981	71	29	17,545	13	87
	F	4,323	50	50	2,255	36	64	22,461	5	95
Austria	M	2,971	90	10	2,236	72	28	33,499	15	85
	F	4,943	54	46	3,226	39	61	56,183	5	95
France	M	1,964	88	12	968	77	23	7,731	18	82
	F	6,421	54	46	2,262	40	60	15,276	7	93
Germany	M	19,629	90	10	11,253	72	28	92,220	16	84
	F	35,710	52	48	17,905	38	62	132,535	7	93
Netherlands	M	3,441	91	9	3,094	70	30	13,111	17	83
	F	3,287	42	58	2,697	27	73	13,672	7	93

incomes and were both more aware and more capable of obtaining good health services, so that they did not need to leave the work force because of impaired health. Another possibility is that their better education led them to more stimulating jobs and careers, and they were less eager to accept early retirement. A third possibility is that, since these countries were three of the four having the greatest likelihood of speaking a language other than English at home, the immigrant groups from these countries were least likely to have job skills and were simultaneously most likely to accept early retirement or have supervisors who encouraged early retirement.

Another interesting observation is that at each age and for each country of birth, far fewer women remained in the work force than men. Approximately one half of these women are in the work force between 55 and 59 years, compared with almost 90% of the men. For the next 5-year span, more than one third of the women and some 70% of the men are still working. By age 65 and over, 15% of the men remain in the work force, whereas only about 5% of the women continue to work. The percentage of drop-off for men is considerably less than for women at each point.

A subsequent statistical analysis indicated the number of women over age 50 who had never had children. These data were derived indirectly from the Census Bureau's special tabulation on the number of children ever born. (This was accomplished by the formula $(M - W)/M$, where M = the average number of children per *mother* and W = the average number of children per *woman*.) Although the estimates by country of birth show considerable variability, a more surprising statistic in our view is that many older French, German, and Austrian immigrant women have never had children of their own.

To summarize the national data just presented: The Euro-American immigrant population as of 1980 was overrepresented by the elderly; among these elderly, women substantially outnumbered men, which meant that most women were not currently married, and most of these were widows. These Euro-American immigrant elderly had little schooling and were very unlikely to remain in the labor market after the age of 65. This was particularly true of women, with half of those in their late 50s still employed compared to slightly more than 5% over age 65 who were still employed.

Now, in order to analyze differences between the old (65–74) and the old-old (75+), we will examine data based on the foreign-born population of New York City.

Demographic Data: The New York City Sample

The second data analysis, conducted from a sample of persons in the New York City area, is based on a limited population, but it offers a much more detailed analysis. This section will be restricted to those Euro-American immigrant groups having a population of at least 2,000 and a high proportion of individuals who depend primarily on a language other than English. Of the 10 countries of birth originally selected, three (Latvia, Lithuania, and Portugal) were subsequently dropped because the number of older persons was too small for adequate analysis.

Table 4.4 indicates that the proportion of elderly among the various Euro-American immigrant populations far exceeds their proportion in the general population—in many instances by three or more times what might be anticipated. Only among Greek and Yugoslavian men and, to a lesser extent, Greek and Yugoslavian women, do the figures come close to the national average. More than half of the Hungarian women, and Polish women and men, are age 65 or older. This certainly supports the idea that these immigrant populations are aging differently from Southeast Asian and Central American immigrant groups, for example. Recent immigration of young persons from these latter areas has provided a very different kind of population pyramid (see Figure 4.1).

Further evidence of the differences for the aging of the Euro-American immigrant populations is found in the numbers and proportions of old and old-old in each of the groups. For example, among the Hungarian, Italian, and Polish communities at least 20% of the entire population is over age 75; the same is true for Romanian women. In some of these immigrant communities the number of old-old persons exceeds the number of those between 65 and 74.

Data on the use of English also deserves attention. Compared with immigrants of all ages, the proportion of elderly who speak a language at home other than English is generally lower, but not much lower. Substantial majorities of the elderly of all three age categories (65–69, 70–74, 75+) and from all seven ethnic groups used a language other than English in their homes. However, substantial minorities, ranging from about 11% of elderly Polish

TABLE 4.4 A Summary Profile of Demographic Characteristics of Selected Euro-American Elderly Groups by Sex and Age: New York City Census, 1980

Birthplace	Sex	Age	Number	% Elderly	Immigration % before '50	% Use Non-English	% Not speaking English well	% Less than high school	% Not in labor force	% Married	% Head or spouse
Czechoslovakia	M	65–69	1020	13.6	43.1	88.2	17.6	47.0	45.1	84.3	98.0
		70–74	840	11.2	59.5	78.6	21.4	35.7	76.2	92.9	100.0
		75+	1020	13.6	74.5	78.4	15.7	56.9	80.4	66.7	88.3
		All	7500	100.0	45.3	79.7	11.5	32.3	32.8	79.5	95.6
	F	65–69	820	9.4	65.9	78.0	12.2	31.7	85.4	58.5	95.0
		70–74	640	7.3	75.0	87.5	21.9	56.3	87.5	50.0	84.4
		75+	1640	18.8	82.9	76.8	13.4	64.7	95.1	20.7	71.9
		All	8740	100.0	58.4	80.3	10.1	35.5	61.6	62.5	91.1
Hungary	M	65–69	1180	12.2	42.4	86.4	15.3	39.0	61.0	81.4	93.2
		70–74	1000	10.4	50.0	86.0	18.0	48.0	64.0	84.0	94.0
		75+	1880	19.5	76.6	62.8	9.6	35.2	84.0	73.4	91.5
		All	9660	100.0	33.5	79.9	10.4	29.0	35.4	76.0	95.7
	F	65–69	1380	10.6	53.6	75.4	21.7	36.2	71.0	49.3	91.3
		70–74	1900	14.5	70.5	81.1	14.7	50.5	86.3	46.3	92.6
		75+	3440	26.3	86.0	70.9	8.7	64.0	95.3	18.6	78.3
		All	13,080	100.0	49.7	81.0	12.5	39.7	67.4	55.0	91.8

Country	Sex	Age	N	%							
Poland	M	65–69	5560	16.1	60.8	72.7	11.2	41.4	51.8	84.9	96.7
		70–74	5460	15.8	76.2	71.1	9.2	55.4	73.6	81.7	96.0
		75+	7460	21.6	90.1	73.2	9.7	59.2	86.6	66.8	87.6
		All	34,500	100.0	57.5	76.6	12.2	41.3	44.6	76.2	92.8
	F	65–69	6580	15.5	80.2	69.0	10.6	42.2	80.9	62.9	95.4
		70–74	6360	14.9	85.5	67.6	7.5	54.7	91.8	38.7	93.4
		75+	11,740	27.6	92.3	76.0	11.1	70.8	96.1	20.3	71.1
		All	42,580	100.0	65.8	76.7	11.9	46.8	72.1	51.8	87.8
Romania	M	65–69	960	12.0	47.9	81.3	18.8	39.6	50.0	85.4	97.9
		70–74	600	7.5	53.3	76.7	16.7	43.4	80.0	70.0	90.0
		75+	1240	15.5	80.6	59.7	17.7	45.2	87.1	64.5	80.6
		All	8,000	100.0	34.5	81.8	13.5	29.8	34.0	72.5	92.9
	F	65–69	740	7.8	56.8	83.8	13.5	35.1	75.7	43.2	91.7
		70–74	820	8.6	68.3	61.0	19.5	46.4	92.7	43.9	80.5
		75+	2120	22.2	84.9	58.5	5.7	54.7	96.2	17.0	71.7
		All	9540	100.0	36.9	81.8	13.0	36.9	62.1	55.3	87.5
Greece	M	65–69	700	3.1	65.7	88.6	37.1	60.0	77.1	80.0	100.0
		70–74	540	2.4	70.4	96.3	29.6	55.6	74.1	81.5	85.2
		75+	1620	7.1	84.0	87.7	13.6	54.3	95.1	67.9	90.2
		All	22,780	100.0	14.7	95.6	24.1	41.8	23.1	68.8	91.4
	F	65–69	800	4.2	42.5	97.5	77.5	80.0	80.0	42.5	75.0
		70–74	840	4.4	59.5	100.0	52.4	73.8	92.9	33.3	73.8
		75+	1320	6.9	86.4	90.9	40.9	84.9	98.5	24.2	66.6
		All	19,220	100.0	16.4	97.0	43.0	54.2	57.6	66.1	87.7

TABLE 4.4 (continued)

Birthplace	Sex	Age	Number	% Elderly	Immigration % before '50	% Use Non-English	% Not speaking English well	% Less than high school	% Not in labor force	% Married	% Head or spouse
Italy	M	65–69	5840	7.7	56.2	79.5	33.9	74.7	72.9	88.7	93.2
		70–74	5460	7.2	74.4	77.7	25.3	75.1	88.6	83.2	93.7
		75+	14,820	19.4	95.4	85.0	21.7	81.4	94.5	64.9	83.6
		All	76,300	100.0	38.4	87.4	22.4	56.9	38.5	74.8	93.0
	F	65–69	7080	8.7	68.1	86.2	35.3	75.4	88.7	54.5	87.1
		70–74	7260	8.9	85.4	85.7	24.8	80.7	94.2	38.6	87.1
		75+	21,080	25.9	94.2	88.9	31.2	84.7	97.2	19.9	69.5
		All	81,400	100.0	48.4	90.6	30.5	65.8	70.7	54.7	86.7
Yugoslavia	M	65–69	380	3.3	63.2	68.4	21.1	57.9	78.9	63.2	94.7
		70–74	320	2.8	68.8	87.5	12.5	68.8	81.3	87.5	87.5
		75+	600	5.2	73.3	93.3	16.7	93.4	96.7	73.3	80.0
		All	11,480	100.0	11.5	92.9	18.6	49.5	19.3	65.7	92.3
	F	65–69	540	4.9	18.5	96.3	40.7	63.0	77.8	40.7	77.7
		70–74	440	4.0	50.0	100.0	40.9	68.2	95.5	50.0	81.9
		75+	820	7.5	46.3	87.8	51.2	78.0	92.7	17.1	58.5
		All	10,920	100.0	10.1	94.5	29.9	54.8	47.7	64.7	87.9

immigrants to more than half of older Greek women, admitted to not being able to speak English well. (Keep in mind that the numbers below the lines in Table 4.4 refer to the entire immigrant population in the indicated category and are not averages of the numbers above them.) While the overall percentage of elderly who speak English at home was very slightly higher than for the entire Euro-American immigrant population, the percentage of elderly who speak English poorly was moderately higher overall than for the non-elderly. For the most part, those over 75 appeared to have greater facility in English than those between 65 and 74.

These data, which appear inconsistent initially, can be explained in several ways. First, it is possible that the old-old, having been in the United States longer (see Table 4.4), have used those years to gain greater proficiency in English. A second explanation is that the old-old may respond to the census questions more in keeping with a melting-pot bias. A third possibility is that the census may undercount the elderly who do not speak or read English well. Finally, among younger elderly there may be those who have arrived much more recently in this country as the elderly dependent of a citizen and, therefore, may not have had the potential and time to gain proficiency.

The measure of level of education for Table 4.4 differs somewhat from the measure used earlier in this chapter. In this instance the percentage less than high school refers to those who did not complete tenth grade, rather than to those who did not complete high school. However, both sets of data indicate that these Euro-American immigrant elderly have had limited formal education. Further, the proportion of those out of the labor force and the proportion presently married parallel the national data. Finally, the great majority live in their own households as either head-of-household or as spouse of the head-of-household.

Tables 4.5 and 4.6 supplement the information provided in Table 4.4. The great majority of older men live in their own homes as head-of-household; older women usually live with their husbands, although with increasing age, they are more likely to be head of their own households due to the incapacitation and eventual death of the husbands. Women are more likely to live with their children than are men, undoubtedly the result of the fact that older men have wives to care for them and older women tend to be widows. Greek and Yugoslavian women and Greek and Italian men are most likely to live with their children. This suggests that cultural differences are an important determinant in this regard.

TABLE 4.5 Living Arrangement of Selected Euro-American Elderly by Age and Sex: New York City Census, 1980

Birthplace	Sex	Age	Number	Percent Distribution					
				HHR	Spouse	Parent	Sibling and other rel.	Inmate	Others*
Czechoslovakia	M	65–69	1,000	96.0	2.0	0.0	0.0	0.0	2.0
		70–74	840	97.6	2.4	0.0	0.0	0.0	0.0
		75+	1,020	86.3	2.0	0.0	7.8	3.9	0.0
	F	65–69	800	35.0	60.0	0.0	2.5	0.0	2.5
		70–74	640	37.5	46.9	0.0	15.7	0.0	0.0
		75+	1,640	51.2	20.7	13.4	7.3	6.1	1.2
Hungary	M	65–69	1,180	89.8	3.4	3.4	1.7	0.0	1.7
		70–74	1,000	94.0	0.0	0.0	0.0	2.0	4.0
		75+	1,880	89.4	2.1	2.1	3.2	2.1	1.1
	F	65–69	1,380	47.8	43.5	5.8	2.8	0.0	0.0
		70–74	1,900	50.5	42.1	1.1	3.2	3.2	0.0
		75+	3,400	62.4	15.9	7.1	6.5	8.2	0.0
Poland	M	65–69	5,540	93.1	3.6	0.4	1.1	0.4	1.5
		70–74	5,460	92.7	3.3	2.2	0.7	0.7	0.4
		75+	7,440	84.1	3.5	3.0	2.1	6.5	0.8
	F	65–69	6,520	35.0	60.4	2.1	1.5	0.6	0.3
		70–74	6,360	59.1	34.3	2.5	1.9	1.9	0.3
		75+	11,720	53.2	17.9	11.4	5.4	11.1	0.8

Romania	M	65–69	940	93.6	4.3	0.0	2.1	0.0	0.0
		70–74	600	90.0	0.0	6.7	0.0	0.0	3.3
		75+	1,240	75.8	4.8	6.5	3.2	8.1	1.6
	F	65–69	720	55.6	36.1	5.6	0.0	2.8	0.0
		70–74	820	36.6	43.9	14.6	2.4	0.0	2.4
		75+	2,120	58.5	13.2	6.6	4.7	16.0	0.9
Greece	M	65–69	700	88.6	11.4	0.0	0.0	0.0	0.0
		70–74	540	77.8	7.4	7.4	3.7	3.7	0.0
		75+	1,620	84.0	6.2	3.7	3.7	1.2	1.2
	F	65–69	800	45.0	30.0	12.5	12.5	0.0	0.0
		70–74	840	47.6	26.2	11.9	14.3	0.0	0.0
		75+	1,320	43.9	22.7	21.2	7.6	4.5	0.0
Italy	M	65–69	5,820	88.7	4.5	3.8	2.7	0.3	0.0
		70–74	5,460	89.7	4.0	2.6	3.3	0.4	0.0
		75+	14,760	80.1	3.5	7.3	5.0	3.3	0.9
	F	65–69	6,980	38.1	49.0	5.7	6.0	0.6	0.6
		70–74	7,240	51.7	35.4	4.7	6.9	1.1	0.3
		75+	21,000	53.2	16.3	14.9	9.8	5.4	0.4
Yugoslavia	M	65–69	380	84.2	10.5	0.0	5.3	0.0	0.0
		70–74	320	87.5	0.0	6.3	0.0	6.3	0.0
		75+	600	80.0	0.0	13.3	0.0	3.3	3.3
	F	65–69	540	37.0	40.7	14.8	7.4	0.0	0.0
		70–74	440	36.4	45.5	4.5	9.1	6.3	0.0
		75+	820	43.9	14.6	29.3	12.2	0.0	0.0

*Others = Roomer + boarder + partner roomate + non-inmate

TABLE 4.6 Poverty Status and Receiving Public Assistance Among Selected Euro-American Elderly: New York City Census, 1980

Birthplace	65–69				70–74				75+			
	Number	% Above*	% Below	% PA	Number	% Above	% Below	% PA	Number	% Above	% Below	% PA
Czechoslovakia	1840	91.3	7.6	1.1	1480	89.2	10.8	2.8	2660	83.5	11.3	2.3
Hungary	2560	89.8	10.2	3.1	2900	86.2	11.0	3.4	5320	83.8	10.2	2.3
Poland	12,140	91.8	7.6	1.2	11,820	86.5	12.0	4.1	19,200	76.7	13.8	3.2
Romania	1700	90.6	8.2	2.4	1420	90.1	9.9	2.8	3360	74.4	11.9	3.0
Greece	1500	82.7	17.3	0.0	1380	84.1	14.5	4.3	2940	78.9	18.4	4.8
Italy	12,920	88.9	10.7	2.9	12,720	86.3	12.9	3.6	35,900	80.0	15.3	4.1
Yugoslavia	920	91.3	8.7	2.2	760	86.8	7.9	2.6	1420	90.1	8.5	2.8

*Percentages do not total 100% due to omission of N/A category (inmate of institution, person in military group quarters or in college dormitory, or unrelated individual under 15 years of age)

Similarly, elderly Polish and Romanian women seem more likely than other groups to live in institutions. This may be a cultural phenomenon or a function of some idiosyncrasy of the New York City population from which our sampling derived.

Financially, older Euro-American immigrants seem to fare reasonably well. In 1981 the proportion of all U.S. elderly living below the poverty line was 15.3%. Except for those elderly who had immigrated from Greece, the percentage of these individuals who lived below the poverty line was considerably less than the national average. On the other hand, the proportions of these Euro-American immigrants who received public assistance for income maintenance was also well below the national average. Since 8.3% of all older persons received Supplemental Security Income (SSI) (Soldo, 1980), these immigrant groups were less than half as likely to receive such income supplements as the general population. This differential could arise from language barriers, lack of knowledge of SSI and other supports, cultural values, or lack of eligibility. It could also arise from an underreporting to the Bureau of the Census, since there was no independent check as to the veracity of the responses.

CONCLUSION

It is obvious from the data that Euro-American immigrant elderly are overrepresented in terms of their proportion of all older people and in their proportion of all Euro-American immigrants. According to 1980 Bureau of Census figures, the total number of immigrants from European countries stood at 4.74 million, with slightly more than 37% or 1.76 million persons being age 65 or older. Of these, a large proportion, half or more for a few countries of birth, are 75 or older. Women, as might be expected, outnumber men. Largely as the result of the substantial numbers of widows, most women are currently unmarried and living in single-person households.

These elderly immigrants had limited formal education, and the majority speak their language of origin at home. A substantial minority stated that they have considerable difficulty in the use of English under any circumstances. Living arrangements were primarily as head-of-household or the spouse of head-of-household, although a significant number of women live with adult children or other relatives. Relatively few had incomes below the poverty line, and fewer still received public assistance.

Prior to the 1980 census, country of origin was asked of first-generation, native-born respondents as well as of those who were foreign-born. These two groups were referred to in combined fashion as the foreign-stock population. The 1980 census dropped the question for first-generation respondents, but it added a question on ethnic origin without regard to the generation or distance from immigrant ancestors. One estimate of the proportion of individuals who would now be considered as foreign stock is that they may constitute as much as 40% of the entire population (Cantor, 1979). The proportion that identifies with one or more ethnic groups is considerably higher than that but, as stated earlier, may be too diluted a form of identification to be useful for a book of this sort. An article by Charles A. Price (1980) may add useful information for interested readers.

In final summary, demographic data can set the stage for the subsequent chapters of this book in much the same fashion as historical background can. Inevitably, not all service providers will find national data useful because many need to develop their plans based on local statistics. In fact, as with most of this book, individual service providers will need to make adaptations to their own communities. Nonetheless, this overview offers a setting and a comparison against which other information can be evaluated.

PART II:
Social
Institutions

5

Families, Assistance, and the Euro-American Elderly

Donald E. Gelfand, Ph.D.

For several decades bemoaning the state of contemporary American families has been a preoccupation of many writers and commentators. They nostalgically refer to the days when the family responsibilities of husbands and wives were clearly differentiated, children were cared for all day in the home, and older parents were cared for by adult children. Surprisingly, however, there has been a growing chorus of praise for the efforts being made by family members today to assist their older parents. The mass media has recently been giving attention to the extensive efforts being made by many families to provide for older persons. The media has also correctly been focusing attention on the emotional and financial costs these efforts may entail for the family. The expanded newspaper, television, and radio coverage reflect an increasingly common situation facing many families whose older members have been fortunate to survive to old age in numbers not thought possible at the turn of the century. It is now, therefore, extremely important for practitioners working with older Euro-Americans to have knowledge about the ways in which different Euro-American groups prefer to assist their older individuals and the approaches these groups actually use.

Unfortunately, our knowledge about family assistance in many of these groups remains extremely limited. Research in the field of

The reactions of Christopher Hayes and Richard Kalish to an earlier draft have been extremely helpful in preparing this chapter.

aging has tended to distinguish only among Whites, Blacks, and Hispanics. In too many instances comparisons are not even made among these three groups. Researchers often present their findings as if all older individuals manifest the same attitudes, values, and behaviors—all derived from one amorphous ethnic group.

A recent bibliography on ethnicity and aging (Murguia, Schultz, Markides, & Janson, 1984) documents the deficient quantity of available material on Euro-American aged. We are fortunate to have some information on a number of groups, but data related to the elderly within many specific Euro-American groups remain almost nonexistent. The danger thus being faced in this article is that of overgeneralizing about the Euro-American family. To avoid this danger, specific references will be made only to groups about whom information is available. As the discussion proceeds, an effort will also be made to highlight areas where our information is weak and needs to be supplemented.

FAMILY STRUCTURE AND ASSISTANCE

Euro-American Family Background

The nineteenth-century European family provides the backdrop for the contemporary Euro-American family. These families had some characteristics similar to those of the modern Euro-American family, but they also had some differences that are important to recognize.

Many present-day Euro-Americans trace their family roots back to the agricultural areas of southern Italy, Greece, Ireland, or Poland, or to the Jewish ghettoes of Russia. In the vast majority of cases these families were large. Children, especially males, were important in working the land and taking care of parents in their old age. Life was difficult, and the family had to band together to survive political changes, drought, and epidemics.

Banfield (1958) has termed the Italian family *amoral,* a term that he used not to mean lack of morality but a strong focus on family survival as the major goal of the family. Indeed, in many countries individual survival was seen as dependent on survival of the family. Howe's (1976) description of the Jewish family in the Russian ghettoes makes this clear: "there was little room for individuality as we have come to understand it, since the community was the manifestation of God's covenant with Israel, as the family was the living core of the community" (p. 13). Cronin's (1970) description of the subjugation of the individual to the interests of the Italian family is very similar. The tradition of arranged marriages can thus be seen as a means of preserving the family by ensuring that the spouse has the wealth or rank to preserve it.

Women and Elderly in the European Ethnic Family

Women and older people had distinct roles and obligations in the ethnic family as it existed in Europe. Life was never easy for ethnic women, and it was made even more difficult because of their inferior status to men. While the birth of a son was celebrated in many cultures, the birth of a daughter was often viewed with alarm because of the need to accumulate a dowry to facilitate the daughter's marriage. As she grew up, a woman learned to comply with the traditional woman's role. In Ireland, this included walking behind men, eating meals after men were finished, helping men with the field work but receiving no help with the strenuous chores of housework and cooking (McCourt, 1979). Added to this was the expectation that women would bear many children because of the low survival of infants.

Women were subject to control not only from their husbands but also from their fathers-in-law. In the European family, authority remained in the hands of the older parent, regardless of the amount of work they contributed to the family or the care they needed. This tradition of respect for and authority of the older person obviously enhanced the later years of the individual.

The tradition was not necessarily seen as positive by the children. Some adult children chafed under the continued domination of older parents. Hostility between parent and child was common in many European homes. In families with a number of sons, the laws of primogeniture meant that only the first-born son inherited property. Younger sons faced difficult times after the parents died. Immigration was seen by many men as a way of improving their propertyless situation. Immigration also improved the situation of many women interested in freeing themselves from the inferior status imposed by the traditional culture. Values do not change quickly, however, even in foreign soil, and the legacy of serfdom (Schooler, 1976) formed the basis for many of the problems and conflicts among families who immigrated to the United States.

It is not difficult to understand the advantages that many family members hoped would result from immigration to the United States, and it is easy to underestimate the hardships and fears that many immigrants had. As Greeley (1972) has noted, these hardships meant that the individuals who attempted the long voyage to the United States were among the most adventurous and self-motivated of their society. Even after they arrived in the United States, the demanding conditions under which they lived were too difficult for many immigrants. The large number of immigrants who returned to Europe are often overlooked (Gutman, 1966). This self-selection process of those who remained accounts, to some extent, for the ability Euro-American families have shown in adapting to American society.

Euro-American Family Structure

The Euro-American family that was transplanted to and thrived in North America is complex even when only husband, wife, and children are considered. Seen in terms of grandchildren, cousins, uncles, aunts, nieces, and nephews, the family becomes even more complex.

In many families there is now an added dimension: a fourth-generation individual. As census data indicate, unless there is a major delay in the age of first marriage for women there will be increasing numbers of Euro-American families composed of parents, children, grandchildren, and great-grandchildren (Gelfand, Olson, & Block, 1978).

What is important about this change is not only the addition of the fourth generation but the fact that each generation naturally has its own set of needs and may look for assistance to one of the other generations. Parents may need and request assistance from their adult children. Adult children may also need and request assistance from their aging parents. Grandchildren may require assistance from parents. Grandparents and the young fourth-generation child may look to the other generations for a variety of forms of assistance. The four generations provide additional resources for the family but also create demands that often seem to threaten family cohesiveness.

The growth of the four-generation family is not the only factor affecting assistance to the older Euro-American. Among the other factors that can be examined are:

1. Where the other family members live.
2. The life situation of the other family members.
3. The past relationships of family members.

FAMILY PROXIMITY AND ASSISTANCE

Although Americans are always portrayed as being on the move to new communities in search of better jobs and environment, it is surprising how many people continue to live in close proximity to family members. In 1981 the Federal Council on Aging estimated that nearly three quarters of all older persons have a child living within an hour's travel time. In the early 1970s a study of Polish and Italian middle-aged men and women in Baltimore found that 70% of the sample had parents living in the same community (Fandetti, 1974). There appear to be, however, some differences in these living patterns among ethnic groups. A study of 386 Polish, Italian, and Irish men and women in the Chicago area discovered that Irish family members lived at a greater distance from each other than family members of the two other groups (Cohler, Lieberman, & Welch, 1976). The older Irish Americans may have experienced the relocation of their children and grand-children, occasionally to other communities and states but more frequently to local suburban areas. The geographic movement of the children may reflect their increased income and education.

Young and middle-aged families are not the only residents of suburbia today. The picture of older people living almost exclusively in the inner city must now be revised. Between 1960 and 1980 the population over the age of 65 living in American central cities increased by 42%, but the number of older people living in the suburbs increased by 90%. In 1980 more than 39% of America's older population lived in a suburban area. In actual numbers there are now more older people living in suburban communities than in the central cities (Fitzpatrick & Logan, 1985). Euro-American elderly are well represented among the suburbanized elderly.

Of course, a substantial proportion of older Euro-Americans live with their children. In Guttmann et al.'s (1979a) research, more than one third of the older Estonians, Jews, and Italians lived with either a spouse or children. The figures were substantially lower for older Greeks and Italians. In California, Cox and Gelfand

(1985) found that 27% of the Portuguese respondents lived with their children. Studying the situation in Ontario, Canada, Gerber (1983) found important differences among various ethnic groups in the proportion of older persons who live with their children.

> Roughly, three quarters of the respondents are still heads or wives in their own homes, while another 11% live as parents or parents-in-law in the homes of their adult children. Clearly, the Italians . . . and the others are most likely to live with their children. Cultural differences may account for much of the variation, but it is likely that the proportion of the very elderly, the sex of the parents, income, language use, and recency of immigration enter into the picture. (p. 65)

Other data provided only a limited amount of additional information because they do not include the ethnic background of the respondents. For example, Cantor (1983), studying the inner city of New York, found that of the 767 Whites among her elderly respondents, 53% of whom were foreign-born, 35% were still living with a spouse. This contrasts with the higher figures found by Gerber (1983) and Guttmann et al. (1979b), but direct comparisons are not possible because of the lack of ethnic identification of Cantor's respondents.

LIFE SITUATIONS AND ASSISTANCE

As mentioned at the outset, the American family has undergone important changes, especially since the end of World War II. Perhaps the most visible change in younger Euro-American families has been the altered status of women in the household. A majority of women now work outside the home at least on a part-time basis. These work obligations may make it difficult to provide older persons with the assistance they need.

It is also evident from demographic data that other siblings may not be available to take up the slack when one adult child is involved in extensive work obligations. This situation occurs because the older person may not have a large number of children available to provide assistance. Families of eight or nine children are less common now than they were in the past. However, there are still differences among Euro-American groups in the size of families. Even as late as 1960 the birth rates among Irish women were higher than those common among many non-Euro-American groups (Blessing, 1980).

Divorce and Assistance

Instability in family membership complicates the relationship between adult children, parents, and parents-in-law. Divorce has perhaps the most negative effect of any voluntary change in family structure (Kalish & Visher, 1981). These negative effects can stem from divorce among adult children or divorce among older parents.

Increased divorce rates in recent years mean that many older people lose contact with daughters-in-law who could provide them with assistance. Even if contact is maintained, adult children who are attempting to meet their responsibilities as single parents may see additional demands for assistance from older parents as an overwhelming burden. Among older parents divorce without remarriage means that many older people have no spouses. If and when remarriage of the older person or adult child takes place, the readjustment of the family relationships can be extremely complex. Remarriage may require adult children to readjust or even relinquish any continuing attachments they may have maintained to former in-laws (Kalish & Visher, 1981).

Intermarriage and Assistance

Adjustments within the family are probably easiest when there is strong agreement on roles and obligations vis-à-vis other family members. These agreements may be threatened by intermarriage between individuals from different ethnic backgrounds. Intermarriage among Whites of differing ethnic backgrounds has become extremely common (Alba & Kessler, 1979), but its overall and long-term effects remain unclear and are often debated. C. Johnson (1985) argues that limiting intermarriage and geographic mobility are vital in preserving the security and status of older Italian Americans within the family.

The roots of intermarriage among Euro-Americans are diverse. Among Greek Americans, intermarriage with other groups was common even before World War II because of a shortage of Greek women (Saloutos, 1980). For Portuguese-American women, marriage outside the Portuguese community provided a method for coping with some of the more disliked traditions of Portuguese culture: "The near tyranny that can be exercised by fathers and brothers over daughters, sisters, and even widows often prompts rebellions: women marry outside the groups and sometimes even outside the church" (Rogers, 1980, p. 816).

If other family members frown on the intermarriage, assistance from them may become difficult to obtain. Older Euro-Americans may also find it hard to adjust to the cultural differences between themselves and their new son-in-law or daughter-in-law, and these problems can escalate into conflict or avoidance. Poor relationships among the family members may become important when the older parent requires assistance.

In order to avoid disagreement with a spouse, intermarried children may attempt to provide assistance to an older parent by using approaches unrelated to traditional cultural patterns. Alternatively, the intermarried couple may attempt to combine the different approaches of their ethnic cultures to family assistance. It is also possible, of course, that the cultural traditions of each of the spouses may dominate in different areas; for example, in financial matters the ethnic culture of the husband will take precedence, while in issues of assistance to older parents the ethnic values of the wife play the dominant role. If the couple adapts to intermarriage by abandoning adherence to any specific ethnic traditions, they may also fail to pass on to their children a strong sense of ethnic identity, including the prescription to provide for older relatives. It is not yet possible to assess the extent to which intermarriage affects older Euro-Americans, but its potential impacts are extensive.

PAST RELATIONSHIPS OF FAMILY MEMBERS

Assistance between generations in the Euro-American family is not only a matter of coping with current situations but is also based on the personal experiences of the individuals. In an extensive case study of four families, Cohler and Grunebaum (1981) argue that relationships between the Italian-American women they examined were determined by the "personality, and by present and previous life experiences of the women within each generation" (p. 334).

Previous life experiences of family members that have included antagonistic relationships between the generations may be carried over as the parent ages and may hamper the development of the assistance needed from children. Past relationships become even more important as the older person's health deteriorates. In a study of Euro-American families, C. Johnson and Catalano (1983) comment, "With the persistence of poor health and dependence

upon others, the patient's mood and satisfaction with social supports decline, and the relationships with the caregivers, in turn,
become characterized by more conflict" (p. 68).

Conflict can hamper not only the development of adequate
assistance from children to parents, but also the development of
strong emotional relationships often labeled under the term of
confidante (Lowenthal & Havens, 1968). Maintaining a confidante
relationship becomes more difficult as a person ages and witnesses
the loss of friends and relatives because of death or relocation.
Faced with these losses, including death of a spouse, the older
parent may hope that an adult child can become a confidante. In
some cases these hopes may be dashed because of poor past
relationships between the child and parent or the child's feeling
that the parent has become too dependent on him/her. This latter
pattern was noted by Simos (1973) in a study of Jewish families.
Among these 50 families in Los Angeles friction occurred when
the parent was seen as overly dependent, or the dependency on a
deceased spouse was transferred to a child unwilling to take on
this supportive role.

Discussion of this potential conflict should not be taken to mean
that positive confidante relationships between parents and children cannot be developed. Krause (1978) investigated three generations of Italian, Jewish, and Slavic women. Her studies show it is
possible for Euro-American family members to serve as con-
fidantes and share the most intimate concerns of the older person.
The importance of the confidante should not be underestimated.
It is often argued that, for the older person, having one individual
able and willing to serve as a confidante is often more important
than having a large number of acquaintances. It is possible, in fact,
that a more positive, intimate relationship will develop after the
parent has retired and has more time to become more involved
with his/her children.

PROVIDING ASSISTANCE TO THE OLDER EURO-AMERICAN

It would be a mistake to assume that family members are normally
performing extensive services for the older person (Arling, 1976).
There is usually little provision of assistance by adult children
unless the older person is seriously ill and needs attention. Until
that time, assistance may include some of the important activities

of daily life such as assistance with shopping or cleaning, but the amount and frequency of assistance will increase with the onset of severe chronic disabilities.

The point at which extensive assistance is required may depend on the expectations of the older person. These expectations vary among ethnic cultures. Elderly Portuguese in California exhibited strong expectations that their children would provide them with extensive assistance, and these expectations were met (Cox & Gelfand, 1985). In contrast, C. Johnson (1985) was surprised to find that 34% of the Italian-American elderly she interviewed in a northeastern city had no expectations of assistance from their children. It is important to know not only what the general level of expectations of parents and children are but also whether the types of assistance each generation expects are in agreement with the expectations of the other. In a study of 90 pairs of Italian mothers and daughters, E. Johnson (1981) found 75% agreement among the sample about advice, emotional support, general availability, and chore help that the two generations should be providing each other.

Expectations can, of course, flow both from parents to children and from children to parents. Adult children may look to older parents for child care assistance, gift giving, and crisis intervention when serious illnesses occur. Financial aid to help meet down payments on homes or automobiles is also a commonly reported form of assistance from older parents to adult children.

The evidence is very strong that mutual assistance continues even as children become adults. Despite what we might expect, the morale of the older parents does not appear to be affected by continuation of assistance to adult children. Lee and Ellithrope (1982) argue that the lack of significant relationships between the giving of assistance and increased morale among older individuals may result from the fact that older parents expect to assist their adult children. In contrast, inability to provide assistance to adult children has been shown to result in lowered morale.

When called on, family members may accept as an obligation the responsibility for providing assistance. Accepting this obligation does not mean that providing assistance is a preferred role. Whatever their preference, it is clear from the research undertaken by Cantor (1979), Frankfather, Smith, and Capers (1979), and Shanas (1979) that the Euro-American family will step into the breach in ways that are remarkable not only for their diversity but also for their intensity.

Cantor's (1979) research in New York City with Whites, Blacks, and Hispanics indicates that the family assists the older person not only in routine activities including cooking and cleaning but also in times of crisis. Shanas (1979) has argued that in many cases the intervention of the family to provide assistance can enable older persons to remain outside of long-term care residences. With increasing recognition of the assistance provided by family members, the myth that the older person will be abandoned by the family should have been dispelled. Recent efforts have concentrated on supporting the family as it attempts to provide for the older person.

If the older person needs a wide variety of assistance during the course of the day and does not live in the immediate vicinity, the Euro-American family may begin to view the necessity of having their parent(s) live with them. Uprooting an older person from his/her environment is usually not a pleasant task. On the one hand, it removes the older person from familiar surroundings and friends. On the other hand, it places the older person in a situation where he/she is not the head of a household. In their children's home any efforts on the part of the parent to assert authority or even autonomy may be unwelcome.

Understanding this, many older parents prefer to remain in their own homes. Finding a means to provide the extensive and intensive assistance often needed by older parents without requiring them to relocate is a problem shared by many adult children. Among the older Italian Americans in C. Johnson's (1985) study, 78% of those not currently living with a child said they would not consider moving into their child's home.

Providers of Support

Although all of the adult children in a family may verbally support the idea of helping their older parent, assistance is rarely shared equally among family members. Research in San Francisco (Lurie, 1978) and Philadelphia (Brody, Poulshock, & Masciocchi, 1978) indicates that there is usually one pivotal person involved in cases where extensive and successful assistance is provided to older individuals.

In the vast majority of cases, women in the family provide the most extensive and intensive assistance to the older person, a throwback to the traditional ethnic family where women took care of the sick and the elderly (McCourt, 1979). Even though they are now actively engaged in paid employment and careers, women continue to be the primary caregivers in the ethnic family. The continuation of this pattern means that some women are now shouldering enormous burdens as family caregivers. Brody (1981) and others have termed the middle-aged women in this role as *women in the middle,* a term that refers to the fact that these women may be meeting the demands for care not only from parents but also from their own children. Added to the complexity of the situation is the fact that, if the women are in their fifties, they may also be facing the psychological and sociological issues inherent in becoming older in American society.

Providing care will be even more difficult for unmarried women because they have fewer socioeconomic resources. As Minkler and Stone (1985) note, this problem is part of the general feminization of poverty in the United States. In many cases the high rate of divorce in recent years means that women will be entering old age without the additional financial resources that can be provided by a spouse. These women are likely to be financially dependent on limited incomes, especially Social Security benefits.

In many Euro-American families, siblings may turn to the unmarried woman, especially if she is not employed, to provide the major share of assistance to the older parents. An interesting case example is provided in a recent popular article exploring the whole issue of care for older parents (Gelman et al., 1985):

> It was her brother Dominic . . . who helped Frances realize that it wasn't just selfishness on the part of her siblings that kept them from helping, but a combination of their own family and job obligations and the natural human tendency to regard an irksome problem as solved once someone else volunteers to deal with it. (p. 63)

A similar pattern can be seen in Sheehan's (1984) detailed description of the problem of an unmarried Irish woman in her sixties with major health problems and meager income attempting to help her mother remain in the community. The very limited assistance provided by a second married daughter living in the suburbs is highlighted by Sheehan.

It is clear that not all children are interested or ready to take on the role of a caregiver. Although the adult child may want continued involvement with the mother or father, he or she may not want to have them living in the same household or to be in contact with them every day.

The same feelings can be found among many older Euro-Americans. They may take on the important task of passing on cultural traditions to their children and grandchildren. When called on, they may assist in baby-sitting or provide financial assistance to their children. Taking on these tasks does not mean that older Euro-Americans do not want to place some limits on family involvements. In her study of older Estonians, Latvians, Lithuanians, Hungarians, and Poles in this country, Mostwin (1979) notes that intimacy at a distance was the preferred choice of the older people interviewed. This pattern was also noted by Lopata (1981) in her examination of older Polish-American women.

By now it should be apparent that there are many unanswered questions about the role of the family in providing assistance to older Euro-Americans. For example, are there differences between Greek and French families in their attitudes toward providing care for an older parent? Are there differences between Hungarian and other Euro-American groups in the extent to which women are expected to shoulder the burden of caregiving, and if so, what is the responsibility of the men in the family? Do women in Estonian-American families have the same caregiver responsibilities as women in German-American families? Do older Lithuanians provide the same assistance to their adult children as other older Euro-American groups? Are the effects of living nearby or at a distance from older parents the same among all Euro-American groups?

Perhaps the most important question is whether the family patterns of relationships between adult children and parents are related to socioeconomic variables, such as education, occupation, and income. In 1979, Cantor found lower levels of assistance from high-socioeconomic-status adult children to older relatives. Perhaps these children had moved farther away from their parents to more affluent neighborhoods as their incomes increased. Perhaps the older relatives had more money, more of their own resources, and less need. With higher income, these adult children may also see other needs as more important than helping their parents. Alternatively, these adult children may resort to using formal services to assist their parents rather than taking on this task themselves.

A comparison of suburban and urban Italians (Gelfand & Fandetti, 1980) indicated a greater willingness of suburban middle-class families to utilize nursing homes for their parents. We can thus expect to find a variety of assistance patterns among Euro-American families.

Based on these and other examples it must be expected that the family patterns of child rearing and assisting parents among second- and third-generation Euro-Americans will not be the same as those among their immigrant forebears: "Family ethnicity emerges no less now than two generations ago from the interaction of tradition and immediate context. For the third generation, that context is radically different from the one their immigrant grandparents knew" (Hareven & Modell, 1980, p. 353). Some indication of the size of the third-generation Euro-American group can be obtained by using Lithuanians as an example. Although approximately 300,000 Lithuanians arrived in the United States between 1860 and 1914, Americans of Lithuanian descent now number more than 1 million individuals (Ališauskas, 1980).

Among older Euro-American immigrants who arrived during the great immigrations of the early 1900s or even the immigration after World War II, a traditional pattern of taking care of one's own may still be in place (Guttmann et al., 1979a). Among recent immigrants from similar ethnic backgrounds, a different attitude toward service utilization may become apparent. A study of recent older Russian-Jewish immigrants (Gelfand, in press) indicates a reliance of these new immigrants on formal services not only for getting settled but also to deal with personal problems. This reliance may be partly based on having grown up under a Soviet regime where dealing with agencies is required to meet all vital needs. The problems that children and other relatives have in meeting their own needs in the new American environment also encourages older Russian Jews to utilize agencies.

Differential attitudes toward utilization of services should alert practitioners to the importance of understanding the diverse attitudes among the wide variety of Euro-American groups in the United States. As Biddle (1981) comments about one group, "Not quite ready to relinquish the familial system of care and yet not always able to pay the costs of in-home and community-based services and residences, American Catholic Irish remain ambivalent and their behavior diverse concerning older adults" (p. 109).

What Biddle (1981) is recognizing is that the ethnic characteristics that often come to be regarded as the heart of an ethnic culture may develop in response to conditions in a new country in which immigrants have settled. The extended family tradition in the United States is not an offshoot of tradition in Italy but a result of *chain* migration to the United States. Chain migration means that after the first immigrants settle in the new country, they send for other family members. Because of this process the extended family members tend to be more closely linked in affection and mutual responsibility than they were in Italy (Cohler & Grunebaum, 1981).

CONCLUSION

Thus, the relationship of older Euro-Americans to their family members is in flux. While older Euro-Americans may be anxious about the movement of their children away from traditional cultural patterns, acculturation to some of these values, including fluency in English, allows the older person to have greater contact with their children and perhaps develop greater intimacy. On the other hand, the movement away from traditional values among some Euro-American groups may mean that families attempt to utilize methods of assisting their parents that are disliked by their older relatives. Balancing traditional family patterns and service needs of the older person are major tasks facing ethnic organizations, service providers, older individuals, and their relatives.

6

The Significance of Neighborhoods in the Lives of the Euro-American Elderly

Richard A. Kalish, Ph.D.

> They left their little village in Russia in 1895: my father, then a two-year-old, his older and younger brothers, and his parents. Their first stop was Manchester, England, where they remained a number of weeks with family members in an ethnic ghetto; then came Dublin and eventually New York City, also for short stays with relatives or one-time fellow townspeople; and finally, Cleveland, Ohio, where my grandfather got a job in a cigar factory. Four cities, three countries, and a cigar factory without leaving behind the ethnic neighborhood, family ties, familiar language, or shared cultural symbols. Each new stop partook so much of the Russian village or shtetl they left behind that, in many ways, the new life was a continuation of the old. And once settled in Cleveland, my grandparents did their best to keep it that way. (Kalish, unpublished reminiscences)

THE NATURE OF ETHNIC NEIGHBORHOODS

What Is the Nature of the Ethnic Neighborhood?

Before discussing the ethnic neighborhood in particular, we need to develop an understanding of what a neighborhood is in general. One authority, in defining *community,* offers what seems to be appropriate criteria for *neighborhood:* a shared geography or territory, a sense of "we-ness" or personal identification, and some form of formal or informal social organization (Ross, 1977). These have been referred to by Gans (1962) as urban villages, when they occur within the boundaries of cities; perhaps they are simply villages when they occur in less populated areas.

To develop further Ross's three elements of neighborhoods: it appears there is a physical or geographical requirement, a psychological or feeling–tone requirement, and a social or organizational requirement. However, these three elements do not operate in isolation from each other, but function as a total system. Any change occurring in one element is likely to precipitate change in the other elements. The presence of all three is necessary to the existence of a true neighborhood, while the absence of any one of the three suggests that what exists is an aggregation of individuals or a group of another sort, such as a university or a shopping center, but not a neighborhood.

Some neighborhoods have distinct geographical boundaries, perhaps a major thoroughfare at one end with a railroad track and a river providing much of the remaining outline. Others blend gradually into other more or less well-defined neighborhoods. The same is true of the psychological and social components of neighborhoods. Some are tightly organized, and a large proportion of inhabitants feel strong neighborhood identification. Others have minimal visible organization and derive little identification. Although they may have a name, they are neighborhoods primarily in terms of geography and facilities, such as shopping centers and transportation networks.

The physical, psychological, or social elements of a neighborhood do not remain static. Housing developments, freeways, business complexes, and zoning changes can alter the geography and thereby the physical elements of the neighborhood. These kinds of changes can have an immediate impact on the feelings that the residents have of living in a neighborhood and of the social organization that exists. Conversely, if the residents cease to feel themselves as being part of a neighborhood because of in-migration and out-migration or other reasons, or if the social organization ceases to function, the geographical area may cease to be an actual neighborhood.

Frequently, several groups occupy a particular geographical area. For example, Black Americans may be moving into an area, eastern European Jews may be leaving slowly, and Ukrainians and a small group of Koreans may be fairly stable. Some facets of the neighborhood serve all four ethnic communities, such as a supermarket, the school, and a fire station, while others serve one of the ethnic groups primarily, for example, churches, a number of restaurants, and specialty shops. This could be considered as one neighborhood with each ethnic group constituting its own ethnic community.

The Importance of the Ethnic Neighborhood

We all live in what can be considered a neighborhood. To a large extent it is within this neighborhood that we shop, go to church, send our children and grandchildren to school, and develop our friendships. We use the neighborhood bar, grocery, pharmacy, and sometimes the neighborhood dentist and physician.

For many Euro-Americans, certainly for those who are elderly today, the ethnic neighborhood is where they went as soon as they cleared the immigration authority. Perhaps they were met by friends or friends of friends, or they just had a name and address on a slip of paper. Perhaps they knew that the neighborhood existed somewhere, and they found it as did the family described in the opening of this chapter. The neighborhood protected them against the shock of having to negotiate their own path through unfamiliar cultures and communities with unfamiliar written and spoken languages.

Many Euro-American elderly have lived in ethnic neighborhoods all of their lives, either in the United States or their homeland. Others may have left for the military, a job, or college, and eventually returned. Sometimes they moved to a suburb that itself became populated largely by that ethnic group. Of those who moved away from an ethnic neighborhood for any number of reasons, some have retained contact with their ethnic group and often with the neighborhood. Others have abandoned their ethnic identification, at least consciously.

Personal identification with the neighborhood, a sense of we-ness, is represented at least in part by feelings of attachment and loyalty to the neighborhood. For many older Euro-Americans the neighborhood is their community and not the larger city within which it exists. Most of the individuals interviewed in Milwaukee by Biegel and Sherman (1979) described their neighborhood as consisting of 10 blocks or fewer. More than one fourth, twice as many elderly as non-elderly, viewed their neighborhood as consisting of only one block.

For older Euro-Americans it is within this neighborhood that they have most of their friends, many family members, and most of their activities. Often they had worked in the neighborhood (especially men, and increasingly women), and their children had been born and reared within the neighborhood. The opening of a new store or a burglary eight blocks away is a neighborhood event. This event is transmitted by whatever written and oral communication nets cover the community. Word of mouth is often the most rapid.

The neighborhood attachment that many Euro-American elderly feel, "especially in urban ethnic communities, provides a sense of belonging, reduces alienation, and enhances ability to solve problems and to maintain the motivation to overcome modern-day frustrations" (Biegel, Naparstek, & Khan, 1982, p. 23). It is also the source of social supports, both formal and informal. These are provided by family members, friends, neighbors, church members, and sometimes even casual acquaintances. Organizational supports are provided by community agencies, often either ethnic organizations or organizations with ethnic leadership (see next chapter for further discussion) or church groups (see "Neighborhood Institutions" for further discussion).

Neighborhood attachment has been defined by Biegel and associates (1982) as consisting not only of attitudinal factors but of behavioral factors as well, including residential stability and home ownership, both of which display a commitment to the neighborhood. These same authors operationalize social supports through three components: direct support (relationships with family, friends, and co-workers), indirect support (interaction with neighbors and participation in organizations), and social adjustment (neighborhood attachment and work satisfaction). Except for the notions of co-workers and work satisfaction, which might need to be replaced by co-participants in activities and satisfaction with personal and social activities, these dimensions seem to fit Euro-American elderly very well.

In addition, these investigators found that neighborhood attachment was more closely related to mental health than either direct or indirect support systems or work satisfaction (Biegel, et al., 1982). Combining this information with the prior studies that have found that the neighborhood is more important to elderly persons than to those of any other age group (for example, Biegel & Sherman, 1979), we inevitably come to the conclusion that the significance of neighborhoods and what happens in neighborhoods have been underestimated in the gerontological literature on ethnic aging and deserve greater attention.

Given the significance of the neighborhood as described above, it is little wonder that Euro-American elderly seem to develop strong neighborhood loyalties and attachments. They tend to remain where they are. Among Guttmann et al.'s (1979a) respondents, who were initially selected because of ethnic identification, almost 75% had lived in the same neighborhood between 6 and 19 years, while another 12% had lived there 20 years or longer.

From the little data that are available, it also seems that Euro-American elderly like the neighborhoods in which they live. Of Guttmann et al.'s (1979a) respondents, 92% said they like their neighborhood. Nearly two out of every three older persons said they felt safe in their neighborhoods.

Comparable data for mixed-ethnic, mixed-age Milwaukee respondents points up how extensive regional differences can be. Largely of southern or eastern European origin, 70% of all respondents, 88% of all elderly respondents, and 97% of all elderly respondents identifying themselves as immigrant or first generation had lived in the neighborhood for 20 years or more. More than three fourths of all respondents were satisfied with their neighborhood, with no indication of age or ethnic differences in this finding (Biegel & Sherman, 1979).

Three groups of individuals are seen as finding their neighborhood of particular importance: the elderly, persons strongly identified with their ethnic community, and lower-income individuals (Biegel et al., 1982). These individuals often find that their major sources of support come from within their neighborhoods. To the extent that these conclusions are valid, it would seem that older Euro-Americans should find their neighborhoods of high importance, since by definition they are elderly and strongly identified with their ethnic communities.

The neighborhood also seems more important for low-income and working-class individuals than for the managerial and professional residents. In his studies in Cleveland, Rosow (1967) found that the elderly who were better off financially and better educated tended to leave the neighborhood for social and other activities, whereas the working class, to which a substantial number of older Euro-Americans belong, found most of their social life in the neighborhood.

Further, for those Euro-American elderly who are most insulated within their own ethnic community, the neighborhood becomes even more significant. Within the neighborhood they know people and are known; they can walk down the street and find someone with whom to talk, who speaks their native language and shares understanding of their ethnic customs. It is where they belong and feel at home, where they probably function most effectively. It is also within the neighborhood where the Euro-American elderly can find a family member, friend, or neighbor to mediate between themselves and the world that lies outside the ethnic community—physically, socially, and psychologically (Berger & Neuhaus, 1977).

Services in the Ethnic Neighborhood

Also, not to be ignored, "People most often turn to relatives, neighbors, friends, and neighborhood institutions for support and emergency assistance" (Biegel & Sherman, 1979, p. 322). All of these serve to decrease the discomforts of vulnerability and increase the overall sense of security for the Euro-American elderly who have remained in their old neighborhoods or relocated to where they have access to these or other developing ethnic neighborhoods. Given such supports within their neighborhood, it has been speculated that these elderly can also adapt to change with less difficulty (Biegel & Sherman, 1979).

For optimum utilization, services need to be located in the neighborhood. In their study of residents of a largely Polish American neighborhood in Milwaukee, Biegel and Sherman (1979) found that two thirds of the respondents stated that they would be more likely to use services if they were located in the neighborhood.

Understanding a neighborhood, especially an ethnic neighborhood, requires viewing it as a system in which all the roles and physical structures—the general and familiar as well as the specific and unique—interplay and in which any change in one aspect of the system also produces changes in the entire system and thereby in each aspect of the system. When the elderly Greek grocer closes his shop, the Italian woman dies, or the Jewish radical becomes more concerned with his health than with social justice, the changes can have effects more far-reaching than anticipated. When people cease to use the subway at night because of fear of criminal victimization, when the new supermarket chain adds a "deli" counter and Abe's Delicatessen closes, when a 70-year-old elementary school is abandoned because there are no longer enough young children in the area, or when the fourplex across the avenue is sold to an extended-family grouping of newly arrived refugees, we know that the elderly will soon feel the impact of the changes.

As these changes affect the physical aspect of the neighborhood, equally or more important they represent changes that will influence the social structure of the area and the sense that the residents have of living in a neighborhood to which they belong, at least in part, because of their ethnicity.

Where Do They Live?

A large proportion of older Euro-Americans reside in urban areas of the Northeast and Midwest. They live in enclaves in such cities as Chicago, Detroit, Cleveland, Boston, Philadelphia, Milwaukee, and, of course, New York City. Some ethnic elderly live in rural areas or small towns, and these are often ignored when considering Euro-American communities. For example, the elderly living in Amish communities stretching from Pennsylvania through Illinois maintain customs and values that are neither German nor mainstream American but are modifications of what these individuals brought with them from Europe (Huntington, 1981). Other Euro-American communities with a rural base include the Finns and the Danes.

The Move to the Suburbs

Initially, most immigrants from eastern and southern Europe located in urban areas, and that is where the best-known ethnic communities and neighborhoods still exist. Over time, many moved out of their initial neighborhoods and established ethnic neighborhoods in less densely populated urban areas and eventually in the suburbs. Guttmann et al. (1979a) determined, at least in the Baltimore area, that some groups of Euro-American elderly lived largely in the suburbs, whereas others remained in Baltimore's central city. Estonian, Latvian, and Greek elderly were among the former; Lithuanian, Italian, and Polish were among the latter.

Most Euro-American elderly, about two of every three, live in a home they own, again according to Guttmann's sample. Once again ethnic group differences are found, and we are uncertain as to whether these differences are idiosyncratic to his respondents or whether they represent national trends. A majority of those whose origins were Estonian, Latvian, Greek, Italian, and Polish owned their own homes, while just over one third of the Jews were homeowners (perhaps because the Jews preferred apartment living).

The assumption that older people live almost exclusively in the inner city must be reconsidered. Between 1960 and 1980 the number of older people living in central cities of America increased by 42%, while the number of older people living in suburbs increased by 90%. By 1980, more than 39% of America's older population lived in a suburban area. In actual numbers, there are now more older people living in suburban communities than in central cities (Fitzpatrick & Logan, 1985), and the Euro-American elderly are well represented among these persons (Gelfand, 1985, personal communication).

In the North, the Euro-American elderly in suburbia represent the aging instead of older people who moved to suburban communities when they were younger and have now grown older in these communities. These communities tend to be lower-income and not characterized by the middle-class affluence usually associated with suburban life. In the South, older people living in suburbs are more likely to be recent "in-migrants" to these communities and to live in more prosperous communities (Fitzpatrick & Logan, 1985).

Sometimes, of course, both the elderly and their adult children live in the same or adjacent suburbs, in which case access of each to the other remains good. Both tradition and practice suggest that it is more common for younger adults to visit the elderly in their family than vice versa, but both practices certainly prevail. Although the automobile would seem to be the major source of transportation for those who live in the suburbs, the availability of good public transit increases the likelihood of exchanging family visits.

In the older and less affluent suburbs where many elderly Euro-Americans reside, public transportation is not readily available. When driving is limited by health factors or financial restrictions, it can become difficult for the older person to shop, visit health facilities, attend senior centers, and return to the urban ethnic neighborhood to visit with family members and old friends who remained there.

For those Euro-American elderly who live in suburbs that have a moderate or high ethnic density, living is not much different than it was in their earlier, central-city ethnic neighborhood. For those who live in suburbs that are more heterogeneous in terms of ethnic distribution, the extent to which they are acculturated can make a major difference. The elderly who are sufficiently acculturated to function effectively in English and in the American bureaucratic structure are likely to find fewer difficulties that result from suburban life than their unacculturated compatriots who may be patronized and disdained as foreigners. However, even the acculturated often suffer from prejudice and discrimination. While both groups may feel isolated from the personal and institutional supports that are so important in ethnic neighborhoods, those who have limited skills in English or difficulty in dealing with the values and expectations of the bureaucracy can find this isolation painful and generally detrimental to their well-being.

In spite of the comments above we do not wish to leave the impression that elderly members of European ethnic communities cannot function without community supports. Most are adaptable individuals who, when necessary, can cope with the mainstream American system without becoming dysfunctional.

Changing Patterns

If there is an out-movement of a particular ethnic community from a neighborhood, it suggests that the neighborhood itself may be in the process of change. When neighborhoods change, it is often the elderly who remain while the young, middle-aged adults, and their children relocate. Over time, of course, many of these elderly die, and leave the survivors increasingly isolated.

As the ethnic constitution of the neighborhood's residents changes, the rest of the neighborhood does also. Churches and ethnically owned businesses either leave or adapt to their intended parishioners/customers to accommodate those who are moving into the neighborhood. Thus, neither the individuals nor the institutional supports remain to provide care, comfort, and familiar ethnic ways to the dwindling number of older Euro-Americans who remain.

In some cases the in-moving ethnic groups become antagonistic to the elderly who stay, and the highly vulnerable older persons become victims of crime or harassment. This serves to increase their sense of isolation and helplessness, which is already strong by virtue of the changes that have occurred and the losses entailed. Therefore, a cycle is established that induces more people to leave and increases the stress on those who remain.

Symbols of the change are the signs in shop windows. For example: A Vietnamese restaurant replaces one pizza place, while another pizzeria just down the street is purchased by a Chinese family. Signs in Greek are replaced by bilingual Greek and English signs and eventually by signs in English only. The small Russian Orthodox church is rented for a Unitarian-Universalist fellowship, while fashionable boutiques appear where hardware stores and liquor stores once did business.

These are only outward manifestations of what has already been taking place. The older Euro-American has already learned that he can no longer take a walk around the block to meet old friends and have a chat. The elderly woman who watched the passing parade from her window has found that not only does she no longer recognize most of the people, but the conversations are in a language she does not comprehend or are filled with so much slang that she is mystified. Further, much of the talk with her friends focuses on who is leaving, where they are going, how well they will do when they get there, and what this means for the neighborhood. When the church decides to move, or when the majority of the congregation speaks Spanish rather than Hungarian, the impact on the older Euro-American can be devastating.

Sometimes those who remain feel like failures: they had not planned ahead for this eventuality; they do not have enough money to move; they do not have children who provide them with the financial and personal help to relocate. As they watch the neighborhood change, they know that with their death their ethnic neighborhood will dwindle further. Thus, they face their own aging with its increased vulnerability and their own death without the care and support of neighbors, friends, and familiar institutions.

Again, it is possible to paint a picture that is unnecessarily bleak. Many of these elderly adapt well to the changes. They make new friends, develop new neighborhood supports, maintain many of the old relationships with those who have moved, and continue to enjoy the old neighborhood with its new faces. The stresses may increase, but they deal effectively with these stresses.

Changing neighborhoods result from a number of factors, sometimes working in concert. One that comes to mind immediately is the deterioration of a neighborhood, perhaps as members of another ethnic group that is less stable financially begin to move in, while the present ethnic group residents struggle to leave. Often this results not only in ethnic differences separating the two groups but also in social class and age differences because the in-movers are more likely to be young, and those who remain are more likely to be old. This creates a situation that is mutually enriching at its best or volatile and hostile at its worst.

A second basis for change is gentrification. The more adventurous young, often with little or no personal ethnic identification, move into a community that has been heavily populated by one or two Euro-American groups. Bases for the sudden popularity of this area with the middle class may be a convenient location, low-cost housing with potential for improvement, or other factors. Now, however, instead of reduced housing prices and deteriorating buildings, the costs of housing rise, and the buildings improve. For those elderly Euro-Americans who own their homes, values rise and the neighborhood improves physically, although it tends to lose its ethnic flavor. For those elderly who rent, housing costs will soar, and they may be forced to move. Sometimes the increased value of the homes leads to substantial increases in property taxes, which also serve to place financial burdens on the elderly who live there.

In addition to deterioration and gentrification, a neighborhood may change its ethnic distribution because a neighboring ethnic community is increasing its population or is pressed by expansion of a downtown area on one border to move in the opposite direction. Although housing costs may not change, the neighborhood becomes ethnically mixed and loses some of its feeling of being a comfortable, familiar, and predictable place to live.

Neighborhoods can also change because the younger people either become upwardly mobile and want larger homes in more expensive areas or simply want to leave a neighborhood where the ethnic density is high. Younger Slovaks, for example, have been observed to move to what have been termed ethnic suburbs (because they have the same ethnic mix as the community left behind) (Stolarik, 1980). When such moves occur, the elderly have the choice of remaining among the new and unfamiliar people and stores or of relocating as their children have done.

Also important in creating neighborhood change is urban renewal: the creation of a freeway through the center of a community, the expansion of a medical center or university, or the reversal of the move to suburbia resulting in the renovation of older buildings on the outskirts of downtown into professional offices.

These changes in the physical elements of a neighborhood will also alter the psychological and social elements. In one city, for example, a freeway made it impossible for residents who live on one side to reach the other side without walking more than a mile. Since many of the older residents did not have access to automobiles and since public transportation was arduous, the neighborhood ceased to be a neighborhood.

Sometimes, of course, when the city itself or professional developers change the physical elements of a neighborhood, they are required to relocate the people living there, often to better accommodations. However, the importance of making certain that the new living arrangements coincide from the point of view of the ethnic backgrounds of those being relocated is seldom considered. The elderly are then moved to a nicer apartment, often in total isolation from their ethnic group.

All in all, it seems that changing neighborhood patterns create greater difficulties for the ethnically identified older residents than for other residents. The more financially, socially, and physically vulnerable the older person is, the more difficulties are created.

Conclusion

There seems little doubt that Euro-American elderly benefit greatly from living in, or having ready access to, a neighborhood where they have friends, neighbors, and family members; and where they feel comfortable, at home, and safe. Further, since many elderly require a variety of kinds of services, there are distinct advantages to offering these services through neighborhood organizations. These advantages include convenience of access; increased likelihood that staff members will understand, and perhaps share, the meaning of the ethnic background; and reduced risk that the older person will get lost in a bureaucratic maze.

Further, close linkages of services to the neighborhood can avoid some unfortunate mistakes. One example is virtually classic. In one Connecticut community, housing provided by the Department of Housing and Urban Development received very little response from Italian-American families who formed one of their major targets. One reason was that the kitchens in these units were extremely small, and the Italian-American families, especially those with elderly members, were accustomed to congregating in the kitchen (F. Rotondaro, personal communication, 1985).

Issues of policy and program development are discussed elsewhere in this volume, and the second part of this chapter will discuss neighborhood institutions. It is hoped that the following anecdote will provide an appropriate transition: An elderly woman who had come to this country from Prague as a young mother just before Hitler took over was leaving her neighborhood to live with her daughter and son-in-law in a suburb several miles away. Much of her old neighborhood had already relocated, largely to the same suburb. In a final coffee klatch, she commented to two lifetime friends she was leaving behind, "Now I will have three neighborhoods—the one where I will live, the one where I will visit you, and the one in my memory."

NEIGHBORHOOD INSTITUTIONS*

Within every neighborhood are many kinds of institutions, ranging from religious and educational to financial and recreational. The specific nature and history of each institution are the result of the unique qualities and history of the Euro-American community or neighborhood within which it is found. Like the institutions of all other groups, each neighborhood institution has qualities that are shared with other Euro-American communities. Some are shared with many other communities in general, and some are unique to the individual Euro-American group under consideration.

In discussing Euro-American neighborhoods we are concerned with three categories of ethnic institutions: those that are specifically ethnic, those that are largely ethnic, and those that are officially non-ethnic but become ethnic as a result of their location. Among the institutions that are specifically ethnic would be ethnic newspapers, self-help organizations, and fraternal and beneficial organizations. For the second category, those that are largely ethnic, we might include businesses that serve the local community such as restaurants; travel agencies; shops that offer food, clothing, or publications directed at the ethnic community; and those banks and savings and loan associations that developed initially to serve the needs of the ethnic community and especially the local ethnic neighborhood.

The third category is also familiar. It includes branches of retail outlets or businesses, such as insurance companies, that are staffed by members of the ethnic community primarily to serve custom-

*For the materials and ideas in this section, we are indebted to the *Harvard Encyclopedia of American Ethnic Groups,* its editors, and its authors.

ers of that community. It provides services, some foods, or jewelry that are particularly attractive to the ethnic community. Another example would be a local elementary school, whether public or religious (excluding the handful of schools that are explicitly directed at ethnic groups). Others in this grouping are libraries, senior centers, political clubs, family businesses not ethnic in nature, and so forth.

Neighborhood Institutions: Past and Present

The kinds of neighborhood institutions in Euro-American communities can be described in many ways. For the present purposes, this author will discuss seven categories, each of which he believes to have a uniquely important place in the history and present circumstances of Euro-American elderly. Sometimes, however, present importance is more a function of history than of contemporary meanings. The categories are fraternal and beneficial associations, boarding homes, grocery stores and saloons, the ethnic press, cultural and artistic organizations, recreational and exercise organizations, and business and financial institutions. We will touch very briefly on educational institutions, health facilities, political organizations, and religious groups, in part because they are discussed elsewhere and in part because their roles are often more familiar and less unique to Euro-American communities.

Fraternal and Beneficial Associations

When the major waves of Euro-American immigration occurred, health insurance, Social Security, and Medicare/Medicaid were unknown in the United States. In their homelands the immigrants had lived in communities where they could receive care from family members and neighbors. As newcomers to the United States, neither family members nor former neighbors were likely to be available for socialization or aid. This was especially true for those who first arrived, and they were usually male, young or early middle-aged, and unaccompanied by family members.

In the event of accidents, illness, or death, these early arrivals had neither the support persons to help them nor the funds to cover the costs of health care or burial. Because any lengthy illness meant additional loss of income, and because jobs were earned and lost at the whim of the employer, income often dropped at the same time that expenses rose.

As a result, these individuals often developed what were termed beneficial associations, frequently at the neighborhood level and sometimes only among a relatively few residents of the neighborhood. Initially, each member would pay a stipulated amount per week or month into the organization's coffers, sometimes as little as 25 cents. Upon need, he (very seldom she) would withdraw what was needed. In effect, they had created a small insurance company from which the members could eventually withdraw in benefits 100% of the aggregated payments. Today's ethnic burial societies, credit unions, savings and loan associations, and social insurance programs are the products of different ethnic communities' responding to these important human needs (Thernstrom et al., 1980).

These associations expanded into fraternal organizations through which members helped each other, and many eventually expanded into social and cultural organizations. Additionally, they offered services to recent immigrants, usually limited to members of their own ethnic groups but not always. Sometimes they would even meet people who had just cleared Ellis Island and other processing stations to offer help. As new immigrants arrived, and as more women, children, and older people joined husbands, fathers, and sons, the associations both enlarged their ability to function as insurance companies and lending agencies, and entered into other activities.

It is difficult today to realize the importance of these associations. Authorities describing such ethnic communities as the Croats ("Croats," 1980), Ukrainians (Magocsi, 1980), and Romanians (Bobango, 1980) as well as others, state that these associations were among the two or three most important institutions for Euro-American neighborhoods. They were overshadowed only by such organizations as the Catholic church.

Virtually every Euro-American community had numerous fraternal and beneficial associations. Among the Italians these mutual benefit societies provided not only insurance and loans but also welfare services that included aid for newly arrived immigrants who needed to cope with physical illness, loneliness, and grief. Provisions for caring for the elderly, especially the ill and disabled, were also found among the Italian societies (Nelli, 1980) as well as among other ethnic communities.

The number of members and chapters was very high for several of the ethnic communities. For the Czechs an estimated 2,500 chapters existed by 1920 (Freeze, 1980); for the Hungarians more than 1,000 such associations were recorded by 1910, with the initial society launched as early as 1882 (Benkart, 1980). Among the Danes only churches and newspapers were begun as early as beneficial societies (Skårdal, 1980). The Lithuanian societies saw their role as extending into morality and behavior since records describe their attempts to keep their members from smoking, spitting, and drunk and disorderly behavior, while also trying to see that they performed required religious duties that included attending church (Ališauskas, 1980). Some Italian societies required their members to attend funerals of fellow members or pay a fine. Hence, each member was not only assured a proper burial but a well-attended funeral.

Over time, the societies within a neighborhood would often merge with other nearby societies representing the same ethnic group, and eventually a national organization would develop. The Polish Highlanders' Alliance was formed in 1927, and the Alliance of Maloposki Clubs, also Polish, was founded in 1929. The Serb National Federation is only one more of many such examples (Petrovich & Halpern, 1980).

The changing age structure of the Euro-American communities also contributed to the development of national organizations. When most members were young and healthy, the pay-in–pay-out structure was successful. As the average age increased and was accompanied by more health problems, the insurance societies had either to reduce benefits or increase premiums. Developing a regional or national base and adopting actuarial practices of other insurance companies were used by some groups, such as the Sons of Italy, to solve the problem.

The membership and power of these organizations, at both local and national levels, have diminished during the past several decades. This is probably due partly to the changing values and options of the second and third generations, who have less need to participate in such organizations, given their access to Social Security, work-related pensions, health insurance plans, and unemployment support from the government and occasionally from unions (Thernstrom et al., 1980).

However, diminishing membership notwithstanding, these organizations still have strong influence in many ethnic communities, and many of them still provide a significant array of services at the neighborhood, local, and national levels. Frequently, the organizations' political strength at the neighborhood level can translate into considerable political and economic influence at the state-legislative level.

Both because of historical involvement and because the elderly tend to remain within the ethnic neighborhood, the services of the ethnic associations are especially valuable to these individuals. Compared to younger residents of these neighborhoods, the Euro-American elderly tend to have problems communicating in English and coping with bureaucracies. These individuals are likely to find information and referral, advocacy, and translation services, among others, very useful. The elderly are also well served by these societies because they are often retired and therefore more responsive to many kinds of daytime programming. Similarly, because the elderly are more likely to have strong ethnic identification, they are more likely to rely on ethnically oriented organizations.

Boarding Houses

As each Euro-American immigration wave began, the first to arrive were men, primarily young and often bachelors. Frequently, those who were married left their wives and children in their home country and brought them over later. Older parents were brought over last, if indeed they were brought over at all, since many preferred to stay where they had lived all of their lives.

In looking for living arrangements, a large percentage of these men selected boarding houses, often owned or managed by a widow or a married couple of their own ethnic group, and not infrequently someone they had known or to whom they had been referred in their community in Europe. These homes offered both room and board in a setting somewhat reminiscent of the extended family. The young men could return from work to a home where their native language was often spoken, a native-language newspaper was available, familiar foods were served, and familiar customs were followed. Boarding houses were common in that era (recall the semiautobiographical writings of Eugene O'Neill and Thomas Wolfe or the comedy *You Can't Take It with You*) and served as a transition for innumerable young, usually male, immigrants.

For Romanian immigrants, boarding houses were considered to be one of the two major institutions for easing the transition from Old World ways to the ways of the New World (Bobango, 1980).

For Croats, one source lists boarding houses as one of the three most important institutions ("Croats," 1980). These are, inevitably, subjective evaluations, but they indicate how important the boarding houses were.

As the institution developed, boarding houses became a major source of income for men who brought their wives over and could afford the initial costs required for the larger homes, although there are instances in which even rented apartments would accommodate one or two boarders. The family that owned and ran the boarding home frequently extended its roles to serve as custodian for savings because trust in local banks was very low, as travel arranger, and as the responsible party for sending money overseas (Thernstrom et al., 1980).

Boarding houses lasted well into the 1930s (Bobango, 1980), and they are very much part of the experience of today's Euro-American elderly. Post-World War II immigrants were fewer in number, relative to the family members available to receive and help them, and they came as family units in many instances. Therefore, the boarding house was no longer as functional as it had been earlier. Nonetheless, it served the Euro-American communities extremely well and is part of the life history of men, now elderly, who arrived between the world wars. The cohort that arrived here when these homes were most significant, that is, prior to World War I, has very few living survivors.

Grocery Stores and Saloons

The neighborhood bar is still an important part of many communities, including Euro-American neighborhoods, where it serves as a place in which people can come together, have a drink, talk with friends, hear gossip from the bartender, read a newspaper, perhaps play a game of chess or dominoes, and feel totally protected. The television show *Fame* provides one example without ethnic linkages; Archie Bunker took over a neighborhood bar after Edith died; and the British version is exemplified in the "Andy Capp" comic strip.

However, the institution does not perform the same functions that it did around the turn of the century. In Polish-American communities the saloonkeeper, along with the grocer, not only provided space for social relaxation but, like the owners of the boarding homes, wrote letters for those not functionally literate, made travel arrangements to bring over family members or to permit the customer to return to the homeland, and performed other related tasks. These individuals were frequently leaders in the benevolent and fraternal societies, and their influence in the neighborhood was far-reaching (Greene, 1980). Comparable roles were provided by saloonkeepers in the Croatian neighborhoods ("Croats," 1980a).

For Euro-American elderly, the ethnic neighborhood bar may no longer provide a resource for writing letters or making travel arrangements, but other resources are now readily available for those who wish help. Bars are still very much in evidence as social and recreational resources—for games, gossip, and relaxation—not unlike their turn-of-the-century predecessors.

Ethnic Media

The ethnic media consist primarily of ethnic press and radio programming. There are also some ethnic programs on television, and some small publishing companies that serve ethnic markets, but these have little impact.

Countless numbers of ethnic newspapers came into being during the late 1800s and early 1900s. Every Euro-American group had at least one, and for more populous groups in larger cities there would be several such newspapers. Although coverage varied, it emphasized activities of the ethnic group and frequently focused on local news. Initially, these were in the native language.

During the past two decades many of these newspapers have ceased publication, and others have divided their copy between English and the native language. This has occurred, at least in part, as the result of second- and third-generation Euro-Americans' having less facility with their language of origin. Nonetheless, these publications are still very influential within the community. They seem to be trusted more and relied on more regarding news of the ethnic community than are the large-circulation newspapers.

Ethnic radio programming, for the most part, consists of regular programming on a local station, perhaps 1 hour per day or per week. The contents of the program, delivered in the native language, would be news of ethnic interest, ethnic music, and discussion of local issues of particular concern and from the point of view of the ethnic community. These programs are most common when ethnic groups, for example the Greek Americans (Saloutos, 1980) or the Ukrainian Americans (Magocsi, 1980), are represented in large numbers.

Although we have referred elsewhere to the importance of word-of-mouth for informing the ethnic community of what is going on, the ethnic media remain very important for informing the community. Its writers and editors know the community and its neighborhoods, its traditions and values, and its people, often personally. They are usually in contact with the changes taking place in the homeland. Most important, they can offer news, issues, local events, and entertainment that are unavailable elsewhere. They are trusted in a way that the non-ethnic media are not.

Cultural Organizations

Many organizations in Euro-American communities were established to provide opportunities for music, dance, and theater. These organizations often attended to the needs of a relatively small membership. There could be several musical groups within one neighborhood, with one focused on singing, another on providing orchestral music, and another on playing for dances. Some performed only for themselves, while others put their skills on display at public performances such as weddings and other celebrations.

These organizations still exist, although in much smaller numbers. Ethnic weddings are no longer as frequent nor as fervent. Ethnic theater is also no longer as familiar, although it has not died out altogether; for example, Yiddish theater is still found in New York City (Goren, 1980), and other examples are scattered around the country.

The popularity of ethnic music and theater during the 1930s and 1940s may be indicated by attendance at an outdoor summer theater in Cleveland Heights, Ohio. During what was usually a 10-week, 10-production season, 3 weeks and 3 productions would be musicals of earlier decades, such as *Sari, Countess Maritza, The Student Prince,* and *New Moon.* Performers in leading roles and choruses in casts that could number as many as 65 or more persons were all local. Dances were frequently performed by local ethnic dance groups. While not all had Euro-American themes, the musical and dramatic style of these productions definitely appealed to members of Cleveland's numerous and large Euro-American communities. The 3,300-seat amphitheater was virtually always sold out for their performances, while the local productions of Broadway plays might attract as few as 200 or 300 persons. Newspaper articles announcing and describing these shows would be provided, in English, to a publishing firm in Cleveland that had them translated and published in some 35 to 45 local Euro-American newspapers. This was still occurring as late as 1948 and 1949.

Certain ethnic groups seemed particularly attracted by certain cultural forms of expression. Thus, music was emphasized for the Germans (Conzen, 1980) and theater for the Jews (Goren, 1980). Nonetheless, there is good reason to believe that all cultural forms were available in most Euro-American communities where the population was large enough to permit it. Euro-American elderly still participate in these cultural activities, and younger people often are active also. Dancing, singing, bands, orchestras, and theater continue to offer vehicles that bring all generations together to participate in ethnically meaningful events.

Recreational and Physical Education Organizations

From early days, many Euro-American neighborhoods would hold picnics to which the entire family would come. The occasions also provided young men and women with a sanctioned opportunity to meet each other or to pursue courtship activities. One description of the Albanian-American community emphasizes that people would travel long distances to attend these affairs ("Albanians," 1980). Festival days, weddings and other celebrations, and U.S. holidays offered additional opportunities to come together socially. To a limited extent, these activities still occur.

Gymnastic societies were also popular. The Czech *sokol* provided one form of ethnically identified exercise and physical activity (Freeze, 1980). Also, the Serbian National Federation encouraged and supported sports and exercise programs (Petrovich & Halpern, 1980).

The Development of National Organizations

Initially, Euro-American organizations were local and served the neighborhood or, at the most, members of the particular ethnic group throughout the city or local area. In time, a national movement began, through integrating various local organizations. These national organizations attempted to bridge not only geographical distances but generational differences. For example, the Croatian Fraternal Union had absorbed other national and local groups by

1925, and it still had a membership in the early 1970s of more than 100,000 ("Croats," 1980a). Similarly, the Serb National Foundation dominated all other Serb organizations and is still successful (Petrovich & Halpern, 1980). Perhaps more remarkable in its way, the Danes have not only maintained the Danish Brotherhood with 150 lodges and a growing membership as late as 1977, but two other Danish-American groups have developed recently, the Danish-American Chamber of Commerce in 1976 and the Danish-American Heritage Association a year later (Skårdal, 1980).

Other Euro-American groups also have national organizations with local chapters, which permit them more power not only for national political influence but also for maintaining a national press and supporting other endeavors at a national level. Older Euro-Americans play a major role in many of these.

Business Organizations

Early in any immigration wave, the new arrivals began to establish businesses to serve the local population. These would include food stores, laundries, barbershops and beauty parlors, pharmacies, travel agencies, bath houses (in earlier times), dry goods outlets, bookstores, banks and other lending organizations, and saloons and restaurants. Banks and lending institutions had their own particular importance because existing banks were often not trusted; nor were they especially interested in serving the new immigrant group which was often viewed as providing too great a financial risk. As members of each Euro-American community became financially able, they often banded together to establish a lending organization of some sort to encourage local ethnic development. The descendants of these organizations still exist.

Neighborhood Social and Health Care Services

We have separated neighborhood services from other ethnic organizations and institutions because we wish to discuss them in greater depth. Additional material will be found in Chapter 7, which discusses the role of religion and the church. Later chapters in this book will be devoted largely to service-related issues. At this point, we will restrict ourselves to a discussion of the relationship of neighborhood services to neighborhood institutions.

Initially, many social and health care services were provided by local churches, beneficial and fraternal societies, and informal support systems. As time went on, areawide or citywide service organizations developed and offered varying services within the ethnic communities and neighborhoods. This is, of course, still occurring, and some of the same issues of misunderstanding are still found. The service providers often do not understand the ethnic culture of the persons they are serving, especially the ways in which the elderly participate in the ethnic culture. The potential service recipients are unfamiliar with what services are available, the meanings of eligibility, how to learn more, and how to adapt what is available to their own needs. At the same time, they may find that their ethnocultural values inhibit their willingness to seek or accept some of the services offered.

Neighborhood services are provided through a variety of formal and informal sources: churches, fraternal and benevolent associations, local businesses, and so forth. In addition, there are the usual public and private sources of services that are not officially connected ethnically but are often staffed by younger members of the ethnic community.

Most probably, the primary sources of help stem from the informal network. Long before retirement existed as a concept and before community programs provided the elderly with services, older people in need were cared for by their family, friends, and neighbors; by their church; and occasionally by other institutions. For many Euro-American elderly these sources of help and support are still viewed as more appropriate than organized services that originate outside the ethnic community. In recent years a substantial literature has developed in gerontological services on improved utilization of the informal network so that its help can be enhanced rather than undermined by more formal services. To a large extent, however, this author sees service providers as continuing to ignore informal supports and preferring to rely on their own capacity to provide what is needed.

Guttmann et al. (1979a) have evidence for the importance of informal services to older Euro-Americans. Of their 720 elderly Euro-American respondents, more than 25% indicated informal supports from their children, and another 29% from friends and neighbors. Since these individuals were essentially functionally autonomous and, for the most part, not in unusual need for services, these findings would be a low estimate for generalizing to the entire population of Euro-American elderly.

Service Utilization

There is a widespread belief and some supporting evidence that Euro-American elderly are underserved in relationship to their needs, in comparison to the elderly of other groups. Guttmann et al.'s (1979a) findings are illustrative. Only 5% of their elderly respondents received help with specific needs from the ethnic community. Of 10 services generally available in the local community, 18% of the elderly received 1 or more of these from the church, while fewer than 10% received any service from other agencies such as visiting nurse services, escort services, homemaking, or counseling. Most services are provided by family members and friends, with agencies and organizations being a poor third and providing only 9% of the elderly Euro-Americans with any services at all.

The research does not indicate whether there are unmet service needs that agencies could provide or whether these needs are being adequately met through other resources. Perhaps both situations can be found, with varying mixes at different times and for various Euro-American communities. Once again a dilemma can be observed. If service providers decide that the informal networks are not doing an adequate job of providing help and support to the elderly, the formal network may step in. This can have the effect of improving available services, but it can also undermine the informal network. The attitude may be, "Don't bother taking Grandma to the doctor's next week—the Family Service social worker will pick her up." The family may thus experience some relief, or a neighbor may spend an extra hour watching television, but the older person may lose some important social time. Conversely, if the service providers assume that the informal network is working, and in fact it is not, the elderly lose again. The need for accurate information is vital.

In explaining the low utilization of neighborhood services, Kolm (1980) offers several hypotheses: first, the Euro-American communities are not, in general, concerned with their elderly and provide very little or no organized support for them; second, since there is a strong traditional belief among many of these ethnic communities that the family members are responsible for the elderly, the ethnic leadership does not assume any responsibility and, in fact, is often unaware of their problems and needs; third, the Euro-American elderly and their close family members are often unaware that relevant services exist and are unwilling to be identified as what they view as welfare recipients; and fourth, agency insensitivity to the needs of the Euro-American elderly clients and the existence of language and cultural barriers combine to keep the elderly from making contacts with what might be appropriate agencies.

It is often stated that community workers are most effective when they involve formal and informal community leaders in their projects and create change strategies that are consistent with the culture of the community (Stuen, 1985). This is most certainly the case with older Euro-Americans. There are existing leaders, formal and informal networks, and values and mores; and ignoring or trying to circumvent these is very likely to be counterproductive.

Inevitably, program planners and administrators who do work through and with the system of people and institutions already in place are required to give up some decision-making power. They also face the possibility of becoming enmeshed in local ethnic–community politics. Thus, there are positive and negative aspects to this form of action, although it seems to this author that concerned agency leadership and planning could circumvent most of the negative aspects. Most certainly, coordinating local ethnic efforts with the corresponding general public agencies would increase the chances of providing effective and culturally relevant services to Euro-American elderly (Kolm, 1980).

Another procedure that will usually improve the ability of non-ethnic service providers to work successfully with the Euro-American elderly is to utilize advisory groups drawn from the ethnic community, preferably including some older persons, and to use local residents as part of the paid staff. Such actions will simultaneously provide a useful source of information concerning the ethnic community and its individual members, and it will also signify to the community that the agency is willing to share its financial resources as well as its expertise with the community. This may also serve to help local people, including the elderly, perceive the agency not just as Lady (or Lord) Bountiful, come to distribute its largesse to the poor, but as an integral component of the ethnic community that operates from inside rather than from outside.

While the general community agencies need to improve their effectiveness, the local ethnic community also needs to participate. "While the ethnic patterns regarding the relations of the elderly to their families should be maintained, the ethnic community should assume more responsibility for their elderly. . . . The community should take direct responsibility for the elderly who have no families or relatives, particularly regarding housing, regular visits, health care, and so forth" (Kolm, 1980, p. 16). (Specific services and programs will be discussed in later chapters as part of a much more comprehensive discussion of services to Euro-American elderly.

The Isolated Elderly

The assumption is often made, by omission more often than commission, that the Euro-American elderly live in communities with high ethnic density or, on the rare occasions when this is not true, are in close and frequent contact with that community. This is not always the case, and many elderly are isolated from their ethnic peers.

This isolation occurs for many reasons. One well-recognized basis for isolation is continuing to reside in a home that has been caught in changing demographic tides and has become engulfed in another ethnic community. This in-moving community may be of lower, higher, or equivalent standard of living, but the difficulties probably become most acute when the behavior and cultural values of the two ethnic communities collide.

Second, those Euro-American elderly who had relocated to the suburbs or who had chosen at some time in their lives to reside in a rural area may find themselves isolated when they become old.

Third, while conversion of a Euro-American group member to another religion is not common, it is certainly far from unknown. The conversion sometimes occurred as the result of out-marriage. At other times it represented an attempt to become assimilated, and obviously many conversions arose from conviction. Conversion was more familiar when two Euro-American groups of different religious affiliations resided in the same or adjacent neighborhoods. Also, those who attended college, who served in the military, or who entered vocational fields that required extensive contact with a mixed ethnic group were more likely to be exposed to the ideas and customs of other religions and were, therefore, more susceptible to conversion. When the converts were already elderly or became elderly, leaving their ethnic church may lead them to believe—rightly or wrongly—that their other ethnic ties need to be diminished or severed. At the same time, they have not established new ties that are comparable.

Sometimes, of course, the individual does not convert to another religion but for philosophical or political reasons leaves the church. We cannot, at this point, describe all possible permutations nor are good data available as to the frequency of conversions or their outcomes. It is simply our intent to describe an event that did occur and that, when it occurred, had significant impact on the lives of those affected. Religious conversion was also a deep concern for all clergy and the devout members of their churches and synagogues.

Changes in Ethnic Institutions

Although there are undoubtedly many kinds of changes in ethnic institutions and the individuals who are most involved in them, we will focus on two such changes: changes in leadership and changes in participation.

Leadership

Leadership of Euro-American communities and institutions is undergoing a transition. In the past, and to some extent today, the leadership is vested in older persons, frequently immigrants or first-generation Americans, who had enough interest in their ethnic communities to invest the time and effort to move into leadership positions. Often these were the individuals who had been instrumental in launching the organizations or in participating in their most significant periods of growth several decades earlier. When they retired from their employment, they had even more time to pursue these endeavors. Now many of these persons have died or are no longer physically capable of maintaining their leadership efforts. Nonetheless, the strong leadership that they have provided has, in some instances, discouraged younger people from being active. As attrition diminishes the power of the old regimes, it is still unknown whether enough younger persons are willing to provide the time and energy necessary to become leaders. The final outcomes—whether a reduced interest in these organizations, the essential maintenance of the status quo, increased vigor with possible new directions, or the creation of new organizations representing a younger constituency—are still unknown.

At this time there seem to be two groupings of Euro-Americans who are willing to provide leadership. One group consists of the more recent, better-educated Euro-American immigrants, who are familiar with the homeland as it was during the postwar period, often continue to speak the language, and are concerned with national social issues. Many of these persons are in managerial and professional categories of occupations. The other grouping is that of grandchildren and, occasionally, children of turn-of-the-century immigrants. In many instances they lack fluency in their native languages, are unfamiliar with their country of origin, and are more concerned with local and neighborhood issues. Fewer of them are in managerial and professional occupations, and more are union members, small-businessmen, and essentially working-class in both their status and their outlooks.

Another grouping of Euro-Americans who seem to have become more active in both ethnic activities and in providing services to the elderly are women of all ages. Paralleling women in this nation in general, they seem to have moved into roles of participation and leadership in many areas of community life and are performing these roles in ways quite unlike those in which their mothers and grandmothers participated in their ethnic communities.

(The statements made in the previous paragraphs are based on informal discussions with members and leaders of various ethnic communities and are not based on careful studies or other sources. Our assumptions are undoubtedly not universal and will apply only in some settings and for some Euro-American groups.)

Earlier leadership often derived from work-related roles. For example, clergy often became leaders, both because of their superior education and because they tended to be trusted by community members. Sometimes leadership devolved on an individual who had begun a beneficial society, a burial society, or some other form of community organization. Those who could serve as intermediaries to the larger surrounding culture—bankers, realtors, travel agents—also might become community leaders (Higham, 1980). Editors and writers for the ethnic press also found a form of leadership in the community.

Higham (1980) has outlined four bases from which he observed leadership evolving. These were (a) providing security and/or needed services for individuals or the community; (b) being instrumental in developing group solidarity; (c) taking an active, perhaps aggressive, position on some form of defense of the homeland; and (d) serving to advance the values, position, or opportunities of the ethnic community.

Participation

It seems likely that the vigor of Euro-American communities has diminished since the peak of the pre-World War II era. Many organizations have ceased to function; noticeable changes occurred during the 1960s. At present, there is insufficient perspective to know whether we are seeing a change in function for Euro-American institutions or a simple reduction in need for them.

It appears that young and middle-aged Euro-Americans do not have the same needs for ethnic organizations as their parents and grandparents felt. Since leadership still resides in elderly men and since these men are often accused of not being sensitive to the issues that their younger colleagues would wish, the latter have dropped away from active membership. At the same time, there is an emergence of middle-aged Euro-American women who are striving for active involvement and eventual leadership. Some of these women arrived after World War II, and some are the grandchildren of earlier arrivals.

As with the present leadership, attrition will alter the constitution of the membership of Euro-American organizations until the present middle-aged become elderly (at which point, those who are now young may launch their own attempts at control). Nonetheless, we need to await the future before we can properly evaluate what will happen with Euro-American organizations.

There has been one kind of change in Euro-American community participation that requires attention. Over the past 20 years or so, there has been a kind of revival of interest in ethnic matters and ethnic origins. The symbol of this revival came from a White-media presentation of Black ethnicity, the television series *Roots,* but the relevant feelings had certainly been near enough the surface to be galvanized by the production. However, even though such revivals are discussed in descriptions of numerous ethnic groups—for example, Italian, Czech, Hungarian, German—there is some question as to both the intensity and the durability of these revivals. First, they are often headed by people who know relatively little of their ethnic history and virtually nothing of their ethnic language; second, they seem to be represented by individual events rather than by a sustained life-style. The response of one author, in discussing the present increase in Oktoberfests, represents this position: "there is little to suggest the renewal of viable German-American culture" (Conzen, 1980, p. 425).

CONCLUSION

To present the views of the author of this chapter: There is little doubt that the contemporary vision is that cultural pluralism or acculturation is preferable to assimilation, and that there is ample reason for ethnic groups, including Euro-American groups, to retain much of their individual uniqueness while also enhancing the capabilities of their membership to function effectively in American society. Newer generations and more recent Euro-American immigrants retain a strong tie to their origins and to many customs and values, but both groups have also done a laudable job of establishing a work life and some personal life in the general culture. Euro-American neighborhoods and neighborhood institutions will not cease to exist, but they will become more acculturated in the same fashion that younger Euro-Americans appear more acculturated than the Euro-American elderly.

7

Religion and the Church

Richard A. Kalish, Ph.D., and Michael A. Creedon, D.S.W.

The three chapters in this part of the book represent, in effect, three aspects of the lives of Euro-American elderly: the family, the community or neighborhood, and the church or synagogue. It is our opinion that these are the most important institutions in the lives of the Euro-American elderly and perhaps in the lives of most of the rest of us also. For the people about whom and, in a way, for whom this book is written, family, community, and church are intertwined. So much of life, so many activities are linked to the church that considering their lives without including the church would be like discussing adolescents without discussing education and the school.

Since the word *church* has various meanings, and since we may shift meanings within this chapter as well as elsewhere in the book, we would like to discuss the ways in which we have used the term. In some instances, church refers to the entire institution at a global level, such as *the school* or *the church;* closely related, the *Church,* by custom will refer to the Roman Catholic church at a global level. On other occasions, the word will have more limited meanings, including those of the individual congregation plus clergy plus physical plant, or only the physical plant itself. The meaning of the term should be recognizable by the context.

Similarly, we use the term *religion* in both global and more restricted ways. Religion is to church as education is to school, or lawmaking is to legislative body. Once again, we assume that the meaning will be evident from the context.

In discussing religion and the church, we have found it useful to use the religious triad (Kalish, 1979) as the basis for organization. Therefore, after a very brief discussion of the historical background of the church in Euro-American neighborhoods and an analysis of the relationship of denomination to national origin, we will examine (a) faith, including values and practices; (b) churches, their buildings and programs; and (c) the clergy and other people who represent the church, the denomination, or the congregation. The chapter will end with some final comments.

IN THE BEGINNING

Virtually all European immigrants had some connection to their religion and to a particular church or congregation (and we will frequently use the term *church* to encompass the synagogue in this chapter) in their homeland. Even those who may not have attended church—the Czech Freethinkers, the unchurched Jews, and the anticlerical Roman Catholics—were rarely unaffected by their religious views and origins.

One way in which an extremely high proportion of immigrants was affected by their religion was as victims of religious prejudice and discrimination. As early as the 1830s, there was considerable evidence of anti-Catholic feeling, and as the number of Catholics and Jews increased among the immigrant population, overt discrimination against both groups was more and more in evidence (Gleason, 1980). When the "no Irish need apply" employment and rental solicitations were made, it was the ethnic issue at the core of the discrimination, but Catholicism was also a factor. Actual religious beliefs or practices were irrelevant: being Irish Catholic or ethnically Jewish was sufficient.

When European immigrants arrived in the United States, they brought with them hope and enthusiasm, but also a myriad of real difficulties caused by the upheaval of migration and the many drastic changes they experienced. Religious institutions, frequently the local parish or congregation, played a central role in fostering assistance both directly and through community networks within ethnic neighborhoods. Conversely, turn-of-the-century immigrants were often loyal to their denominations and to the local church or synagogue. They would pool their money and skills to build a church as their contribution to the religious–ethnic community and to their God.

Much of the life of the community revolved around the church: ceremonies and rituals such as weddings, funerals, christenings, and bar-mitzvahs; many festivals, holidays, and communitywide celebrations, including occasions that celebrated events from the homeland; social service and some recreational activities; volunteer work for the community or the church; and, of course, matters of spiritual well-being. In spite of the numerous neighborhood associations and organizations, the church was often the most important and influential institution in the community and provided important linkages among the other institutions.

Even today, the church is likely to be the hub of the ethnic neighborhood. However, in addition to recent and ongoing changes created by acculturation, assimilation, out-marriage, relocation, and so forth, we also need to examine the characteristics of recent immigrant groups. It may well be that time of arrival in this country is a more powerful determinant of religious values and affiliations than the nation or region from which they arrived. For example, recent immigrants from eastern Europe have lived under communism their entire lives, and they may have a very different sense of religious identity and values than do those elderly who came to this country as children, even when both groups are, at least nominally, Roman Catholic or Jewish.

Two groups come to mind in this regard: Hungarian freedom fighters who arrived here in the late 1950s may have very different religious views from those of the Hungarians who immigrated prior to World War II, even though of the same chronological age. Those Russian Jews who immigrated primarily within the last 10 or 15 years, many of whom reside in Brooklyn, may be very different in religious values or practices from their Jewish neighbors a mile away.

RELATIONSHIP OF DENOMINATION TO NATIONAL ORIGIN

The assumption is often made that each ethnic group is related, virtually one to one, to a religious denomination. This may be true in some instances but inaccurate in others. In fact, religious divisions within an ethnic community or neighborhood sometimes create what amounts to two ethnic groups, while in other instances the differences are readily bridged.

Data are often not available in this regard. The Bureau of Census, by law, cannot ask questions about religious beliefs or denominational affiliation; denominations, by inclination, tend not to ask questions about national origin. As a result we have two sets of data, one gathered by government and pertaining to national origin and the other gathered by denominations and pertaining to affiliation. Data about religious beliefs tend to come from Gallup or other polls or academic surveys.

Thus, we make assumptions, probably accurate for the most part, about the distribution by nationality for denominations or by denomination for national origins. In doing so, several permutations are possible. One occurs when national origin and denomination are identical. For example, most older Greek immigrants and those descendants who maintain strong ethnic identification would presumably be affiliated with the Greek Orthodox church; conversely, most members of the Greek Orthodox church are of Greek origin. In fact, Guttmann et al. (1979a) confirm this: of the elderly Greek Americans they interviewed, 99% were Greek Orthodox.

The second category consists of situations in which national origin is predictive of denomination, but denomination does not predict national origin. For example, 99% of the Italian-American elderly interviewed by Guttmann et al. (1979) were Roman Catholics, but most Roman Catholics have national origins other than Italian; and therefore, in some locales any one ethnic group will constitute only a minority of the members of a Roman Catholic congregation. This suggests that a Greek Orthodox man or woman can attend church almost anywhere and know that the congregation will be primarily of Greek ancestry; the Italian-American man or woman does not share this.

This is true not only for the Roman Catholics but for other denominations as well. Again referring to Guttmann et al.'s data, 89% of the Estonian elderly and 94% of the Latvian elderly are Lutheran, but large proportions of Germans and Swedes are also Lutheran.

A third category occurs when national origin is not predictive of religious denomination. In Germany and the Netherlands, Protestants predominate in the northern sections of the country, while Catholics are more numerous in the south. The same is relatively true for Italy. Since immigration does not occur randomly throughout a nation but tends to take place from certain regions, immigrants in the United States from these countries may not represent the population of the entire nation. Thus, virtually all of the Italians who came to the United States were from Catholic sections of Italy (Pasquariello, 1979).

Another example is that of the Hungarians. Guttmann et al. (1979a) found that 58% of those interviewed were Roman Catholic, while 20% were Reformist Calvinist, and another 11% were Jews. Although these figures are undoubtedly the result of his procedures in selecting respondents (referred by community institutions and leaders), they also reaffirm the hazards of assuming that denomination is fully predictable from national origin.

A final category is that of minority religious groups or denominations that are found in numerous countries. This describes the Jews in particular, although not exclusively. Interestingly enough, Guttmann et al. found that some 7% of those who were referred to them as elderly ethnic Jews stated either another religion or no religion in the interview.

It is important to note that religious institutions and ethnic associations, organizations, and societies are not as closely related and compatible as is often believed. In fact, religious associations have often splintered an ethnic community along denominational lines and have thereby limited the ability of the community to press for collective action to gain goals in the larger community. For example, a typical Slovak-American neighborhood may have three or four congregations, often with little communication among them (Thernstrom et al., 1980).

Similarly, Czech Freethinkers and the Czech Roman Catholics differ greatly on the issue of support for public versus parochial schools (Freeze, 1980). A German-American Catholic may live next door to a German-American Lutheran; while they will be cordial, exchange greetings, and perhaps provide neighborly acts for each other, they will seldom if ever attend each other's lodge or social functions. Ethnic groups that are very small in number will seldom be able to establish their own churches and are limited to being minorities even within their congregations (Thernstrom et al., 1980).

In examining the relationships between national origin and religious denomination, a number of questions arise. First, are ties to religion stronger than ties to ethnicity? Does this vary from nation to nation, or in some instances from region to region within nations, in predictable ways? How strong are regional ties in comparison to national ties—for example, northern versus southern Italy, urban versus rural Lithuania? How significant is language in binding people of different regions or different religions together? What happens when language ties cross national ties? How significant is language, including dialects, in establishing regional or religious differences?

FAITH, VALUES, AND PRACTICES

The first component of the religious triad is faith, which for our purposes will be defined as including religious values and practices. We will also include religious feelings, experiences, and knowledge. These factors are drawn in large part from the seminal work of sociologist Charles Glock (Glock & Stark, 1965) and its applications to the elderly (Moberg, 1971). Glock developed four dimensions of religiousness, with a fifth dimension that he viewed as cutting across the other four. The dimensions were religious beliefs (ideological), religious practices (ritualistic), religious feelings (experiential), and religious knowledge (intellectual); the final dimension was how people behaved as a result of their espoused religion.

Religious Beliefs

There is little doubt that the elderly value their religion immensely. More than 80% agree that their faith is the most important influence in their lives (Princeton Religion Research Center, 1982), and research indicates that older people are more likely to believe in God and in the traditional view of life after death than are the non-elderly (Moberg, 1971). Do the generational differences in these and other religious beliefs arise from age-cohort differences or from developmental differences? That is, do older people hold to more traditional religious beliefs because of their early socialization and religious standing; or because of the aging process itself, perhaps their increasing closeness to death, which creates circumstances that give more credence to these beliefs? Perhaps both factors are operating. There is no evidence to answer this question, but we tend to favor the age-cohort effect as the more significant factor, with the development effect as secondary.

Comparable studies of Euro-American elderly are lacking, although numerous written sources acknowledge them as, for the most part, deeply religious. Thus, the Italian Americans are described as very pious and therefore religious. They are in constant dialogue with God and God's world (Pasquariello, 1979). The contents of religious beliefs of the Euro-American elderly, as well as the intensity, vary greatly as a function of denominational affiliation, identification, and unique personal qualities. From godless atheism to the most fundamentalist Catholic and Protestant beliefs and Orthodox Judaism, older Euro-Americans can be found at all points on the continuum. However, it is commonly assumed that those individuals with strong ethnic ties also have strong ties to the belief systems of the denomination (or, in some instances, one of the denominations) of their ethnic community.

We agree with this assumption, and since older people were for the most part socialized in their childhood to what is now viewed as more traditional beliefs, we also assume that older Euro-Americans have more traditional belief systems than their non-elderly ethnic counterparts. Nonetheless, there are Euro-American elderly who maintain strong ethnic ties but do not attend church nor subscribe to the usual religious beliefs. It would be interesting to know who these people are and how they fit into their ethnic communities.

Religious Practices

Religious ceremonies and rituals can be practiced at home, either with others or alone, and in a church setting usually, but not necessarily, with others. People can also find other settings if they wish. Prayer and Bible reading are frequently home-centered activities, often performed alone. Older people, in part because of their difficulty in getting to church and in part because of individual preference, participate more in these activities than do the non-elderly (Finney & Lee, 1977).

Data for the general population shows that those over 65 have slightly higher church attendance than those under 65 (Harris & Associates, 1975); another source confirms this, indicating that an average of 49% of older persons attend church weekly, a figure that is higher than for any other age group (Princeton Religion Research Center, 1982). When viewing religious services on television is included, the differences between the elderly and non-elderly become even greater (Moberg, 1971).

Limited information for Euro-American elderly is available, based on the extensive work of Guttmann et al. (1979a). More than 80% of their Polish-American respondents said that they attended church frequently, as did about 75% of the Greek Ameri-

cans and nearly 70% of the Lithuanians. On the other hand, just
over one third of the Jewish and Latvian elderly claimed frequent
attendance. The older Jews were also lowest (55%) in stating that
they belonged to a congregation, while more than 90% of the
Estonians, Latvians, Greeks, and Poles stated such affiliation.
However, the Polish Americans interviewed in the Baltimore area
differed so greatly from those interviewed in the Washington, DC,
area on this question, that we need to continue reminding ourselves of regional variations within Euro-American communities
on this and other issues.

Many, perhaps most, older Euro-Americans have roots that are
deeply planted in the community in which they live and in the
church that they attend. This means that they probably have
friendships that date back many decades, often to the town in the
"old country" where the friendship began. Since so much is
shared—ethnicity, church membership, history after arriving in
the United States, neighborhood, language—church members
form a natural, informal support group in general and when troubles occur. On occasion these support groups may become formalized, as when an elderly person becomes incapacitated and the
members of the congregation plan a program of care with home-
cooked meals, housecleaning, and so forth. For the most part, this
is not the case, and the support group functions informally.

Since church services are obviously important to older persons,
are individual churches that serve older Euro-Americans doing
anything to enable these individuals to participate? The answer is
definitely affirmative. Some churches provide transportation to
services for those elderly who cannot get there without such help.
Clergy often visit the homebound and institutionalized elderly.
For those churches that have enough elderly members who prefer
a language other than English, services are sometimes provided in
that language on a regular basis, weekly if warranted, less frequently if not. Of those interviewed by Guttmann et al. (1979a), 29%
stated that their churches offered services in their native language,
and another 29% reported a combination of English and their
native language. Of the Estonians, Latvians, and Greeks, more than
90% indicated that some or all of the services they attended were
in their native language.

In addition to the regular church services, some congregations
provide celebrations of festivals and saints' days that were traditionally performed in the "old country." They also may offer the
Christmas and Easter rites that were performed in the European

homelands. On those occasions when local communities set up ethnic festivals and invite all interested groups to participate, it is often the churches that provide the ideas and the organizers to make the festivals possible. Indeed, almost every ethnically dominated parish in a Connecticut survey had such events (Creedon, in preparation).

Although neither church services nor holiday celebrations are specifically for the elderly, they often depend greatly on the elderly, both as audience and as active participants. Nor is it unusual for people of the ethnic community to come from great distances to watch and participate. Obviously, some people not of the ethnic group come for enjoyment and to learn about ethnic customs; but the meaning for members of the ethnic community, and most certainly for older members of these communities, is very different. Even when an outside observer might view them as effectively assimilated, the call of a service in Slavic, a Greek Easter celebration, or a reasonably traditional Oktoberfest may touch the chord necessary to bring some people many miles.

Religious Feelings

It is difficult to know whether older people are more likely to have religious feelings and experiences than the non-elderly. Moberg's review (1971) of the literature identifies two studies in which this does occur and no studies with contrary results, but Moberg himself is extremely cautious in his own conclusions. There is, to our knowledge, absolutely nothing that systematically examines the religious feelings or experiences of older Euro-Americans, and therefore, like Moberg, we will leave this issue open-ended.

Religious Knowledge

Once again Moberg (1971) has concluded from a review of the literature that we cannot adequately compare the religious knowledge of the elderly and non-elderly. Apparently it is a function of the particular group of elderly, the extent of their education and religious involvement, and the nature of the knowledge or information that is sought. We believe that we can make similar assumptions about Euro-American elderly, in comparison with both Euro-American non-elderly and those elderly who are not Euro-American. Evidence is totally lacking, and we will accept the fact that we just do not know.

CHURCHES AND PROGRAMS

Churches and church-related programs are a form of representation of values and beliefs, placed out in the real world where they can have an impact on real people. For this chapter, we will discuss the following concerns: sense of group identity, physical plant, and church services provided.

Sense of Group Identity

The sense of belonging is a vitally important requirement of personal and spiritual well-being. It is represented in Maslow's hierarchy of needs along with love, and it is similarly represented in Murray's needs as the "need for affiliation" (Maslow, 1970; Murray, 1938). For the older European immigrant as well as for many others, the church provides both a physical place and a group of people that offer a sense of belonging and group identity. The church is a link with the past and the older person's forebears, as well as with the future and his/her descendants. It connects the elderly individual with family members and co-religionists elsewhere in the world, and it provides ongoing relationships. The building itself is part of this group identity: it is a kind of home, familiar and known.

If the particular congregation—or for some like the Greek Orthodox and the Jews, the entire denomination—is linked closely to a single ethnicity, the sense of belonging is likely to become more intense. Also, in many instances the older person has made most of his/her friends among other members of the congregation, and they share a common history. If a common, non-English language is also shared, it is probable that the sense of belonging becomes even stronger. Not to be ignored is the possibility that older Euro-Americans living in a particular few-block area of Cleveland, Pittsburgh, Boston, or San Francisco may have lived in the same community in Estonia, Germany, Ireland, or Russia. If that older person visits another city and attends a church of his/her denomination that is attuned to his ethnicity, he/she is likely to feel at home there as well.

The sense of belonging and group identity offered by the ethnic church is often overlooked. We believe, although we have no empirical evidence, that the church provides this function more effectively for older Euro-Americans than for urban elderly in general.

Physical Plant

Churches offer a place that is frequently available for a variety of activities for older people. In many instances they offer the only place that can be used during those hours when businesses, government offices, schools, and colleges are operating at full capacity.

We mentioned above that churches are like home to many people, which means that others may view them as someone else's turf and therefore to be avoided. An elderly Jew who escaped from Poland just before World War II might not find a Polish Catholic Church a place that he/she would like to visit, or the opposite may be the case.

Regardless of what outsiders may think of a particular church, the elderly who attend the church or who are comfortable there will come much more readily to the church for activities than to alternative physical facilities if any exist.

Services Provided

The basic role of the local congregation in ministering to the elderly is very significant but often vague. Some denominations, such as the Church of the Latter-Day Saints, have a philosophy that requires the congregation to provide comprehensive services to its members in need. Other denominations view the role of the congregation as providing for worship and personal relationships, but not extending to services and programs.

Several questions arise in this regard. What, if any, services are to be offered? To whom? How will they be financed? How will they be staffed? How much religious content will be incorporated? At what organizational level within the denomination will the services be offered?

The first question is, in many ways, the most easily answered: "It depends." Many congregations, including those of Euro-American membership, offer such basic programs as friendly visitors and transportation to church services. These are readily extended to transportation to other resources, for example, physician's office, shopping, barbershop or beauty shop, or to providing meeting rooms for organized groups of older persons. Larger and wealthier congregations can, of course, offer a greater variety of services and reach more older people. Both smaller and larger congregations can deal with their individual limitations by banding together in ecumenical groups to provide services that could not be provided by any one or two working autonomously. The particular services offered are often selected as the result of one or two forceful advocates or a suggestion, perhaps with the "carrot" of funds to back it up, by the local Area Agency on Aging. There are so many services needed and so few provided that developing priorities on rational grounds can be very difficult.

The potential recipients of the service need to be selected on the basis of a policy developed and agreed to by appropriate decision-makers. The congregations need to decide on the geographical boundaries within which they will offer the services and to select recipients. They need to have a clear statement as to the psychological, medical, social, and financial characteristics that qualify someone to receive services. They also need to come to an agreement as to which demographic characteristics fall within their limits, with particular attention to the ethnicity and denominational affiliation of the recipients. A church may decide to include only its members, all local members of the denomination whether church members or not, all local or nonlocal members of the targeted ethnic group or groups, or anyone, without regard to religious affiliation or ethnic membership. Each of these populations has its pros and cons, but the need for a clear statement of policy for participants is incontrovertible. It can be changed later if it proves not to be feasible.

Our present concern with financing and staffing is limited to the degree to which money will be raised and staff will be recruited from people of the targeted ethnic group and from either the local congregational roster or the religious denomination represented by the church. The pros and cons to any position that is selected are considerable.

The extent to which religious content will be incorporated into the program and exactly how it will be incorporated, will be determined to a large degree by the way the previous three questions are answered: who receives the services, who funds the services, and who staffs the programs.

Finally, at what organizational level will the service be offered? By the congregation? The diocese or smaller region? The larger region? Administratively unconnected with any of the churches? For example, the Jewish community has a long tradition of service to the elderly with the great majority of professional services being provided by organizations that are obviously Jewish and under the leadership of members of the Jewish community but conducted by service agencies unrelated to any of the synagogues. Catholic social services may bear a similar relationship to individual Catholic churches even though the service agency is clearly affiliated to the Church on the diocesan level.

Having touched a few paragraphs ago on the issues that arise in determining which services to offer, we can now make some specific suggestions that can be considered only after a sound policy regarding the above concerns has been outlined. These services seem highly appropriate for church-related groups to undertake: outreach to the homebound and institutionalized elderly, escort and transportation services, mobile meals, telephone reassurance, day care for the ambulatory, recreation, adult education, senior clubs, some information and referral, organized tours and visits (for example, to museums, athletic events, and overnight vacations), crisis work, housing, personal advocacy in health settings, friendly-visitor programs, Bible reading, foster grandparent programs, and religious discussion groups. This is far from a comprehensive list and is culled from a variety of sources.

All of the above services and many others are now being conducted at churches around the country. Traditionally, churches have established friendly-visitor programs and socializing opportunities for the healthy elderly. However, many of the programs described above require formal organization and physical facilities, and they are not currently available through churches in many communities.

A recent research finding deserves attention before this section is completed. In a preliminary study of services provided to the elderly by Euro-American congregations in the Bridgeport, Connecticut, area, it was learned that each of the 15 churches that responded had established operations to visit those who were confined, temporarily or permanently, to their homes. The visitation committees consisted of 4 to 25 persons, and those who received visits were predominantly elderly. Those established through Roman Catholic parishes had been developed within the previous 10 years and thus represent a major expansion of the Church's outreach to the frail elderly. Attempts are made to match the visitor with the person visited in terms of ethnic background and language spoken, particularly when the homebound have significant difficulty in speaking English (Creedon, in preparation).

CLERGY

The third component of the triad is the clergy, along with other church-related persons such as religious social workers, recreation administrators, education directors, and so forth. Of these, the clergy remain the focal point.

The graying of America is probably occurring more rapidly in religious institutions than in the country as a whole. The average age of members of many congregations is rising. In part this represents the general aging of the nation, but in part it also represents the unwillingness of younger people to affiliate with mainstream religions. Moberg (1983) cites a Presbyterian publication to the effect that over 40% of denominations such as the Christian Church (Disciples of Christ) and Presbyterian Church are over age 55.

An understandable response of both the clergy and the congregational leaders is to develop programs to bring in more young members, but in so doing they often ignore the growing proportion of their membership that is elderly or approaching retirement age.

In the Roman Catholic Church, the mean age of priests and sisters is also rising. In some orders of sisters, one third to one half or more of their membership is in their sixties or older, and younger women are not entering the orders in large numbers. To the best of our knowledge it is believed that the mean age of mainstream Protestant ministers is also increasing.

There is no doubt that the clergy play a central role in guiding the policy of their churches and synagogues and of their denominations regarding the role of the elderly. No matter how well trained a lay member of the congregation might be, there are many occasions when only the minister, priest, or rabbi will suffice.

The roles of the clergy are many, but five stand out as having particular relevance for the elderly: worship leader, counselor, organizer, advocate, and educator.

Worship Leader

In the role of worship leader, the clergy conduct the weekly service, prepare and deliver sermons, and perform sacramental rites. Those pastors who can speak the ethnic language can offer worship in the native tongue of some of their parishioners, and among Roman Catholics they can take confessions in the same language. Even if only a small proportion of the congregation uses a non-English language, the pastor can offer at least an occasional service for those individuals if he can also speak that language. One New England parish, for example, offers mass in Italian once a month even though only 5% of the parishioners are first-generation Italian (Creedon, in preparation).

Counselor

It is well known that a significant role for all clergy is that of counselor. For older Euro-Americans, the priest or minister becomes even more important than for their younger compatriots and their second-generation age peers. These Euro-Americans grew up in societies in which psychologists and psychiatrists were only for crazy people. The priest was the wise and educated man who had traveled and been permitted experiences that the life circumstances of most of these individuals prohibited. One can go to a priest or minister with troubles, especially if he (almost never *she* for these people) shares cultural and ethnic background and language. In doing so one was certain of being understood, retaining privacy, and having a moral and God-inspired basis for the counsel and advice or for whatever process the priest used in his counseling.

In spite of the relatively benign meaning of going to a clergyman for help, many elderly Euro-Americans will not seek such help directly. Their children often approach the priest, minister, or rabbi, and the eventual counsel or help is provided indirectly, as though by accident, almost as though acceptance were a favor to the pastor. Much geriatric counseling by pastors, at least according to recent preliminary findings, concerns intergenerational issues, perhaps reflecting the differing levels of acculturation and assimilation of the elderly Euro-Americans and their first- and second-generation descendants.

The general acceptability of pastors as counselors leads professional staff at agencies to enlist their help with elderly persons. Calls come to pastors from nurses, police, hospital staff, and other service providers, asking that they see a particular elderly person of their own ethnicity or an ethnic group that is well-represented in their congregation. The issue may be language or culture or the credibility that many older Euro-Americans attribute to pastors.

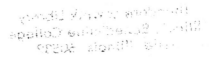

Conversely, since clergy are seldom trained in counseling the elderly, they will also refer some of their older members to community-based professionals. This tends to occur when the issues are more serious, such as severe and chronic depression or dealing with a family member who has Alzheimer's disease. In the Connecticut study (Creedon, in preparation), for example, Roman Catholic pastors readily mention Catholic Charities as a source of counseling and other services, but they sometimes ignore other service resources.

Whether they like it or not, whether they feel capable or not, Euro-American clergy are going to be sought as counselors for elderly parishioners, and they can both provide counsel and refer those individuals who need the help of others. However, this requires that they receive some training in psychological, sociological, and health-related aspects of aging and that they become aware of effective community resources and professional services.

Organizer

The organization of parish services for the elderly is dependent in large measure on the willingness, initiative, and follow-through of the pastor. Although women religious, permanent deacons, and lay committees are often formally responsible for the organized services to older people, it is frequently the leadership and organizational ability of the pastor that determine whether the services are effectively carried out.

Advocate

Clergy can serve as advocates for the elderly in a variety of ways. First, of course, they can represent the elderly to others in the congregation and to those who make denominational decisions at the local and regional levels; second, they can advocate improved services and improved human responsiveness for older persons in legislative and other governmental bodies; third, they can present the case for the elderly to religious and other leaders at the national and, if relevant, international levels.

In addition, clergy can serve as advocates for older Euro-Americans in a very specific way. It is not unusual for younger family members to deprecate the use of traditional practices—the native language and other vestiges of the country of origin. The clergy can represent the older person by supporting these actions in discussions with younger family members, in terms of both their significance to the older individual and their importance in maintaining the status of the ethnic group.

There are also occasions when a particular elderly individual needs someone to help obtain services. In many such instances, the appearance of, or even a telephone call from, a local pastor may bring results more quickly than contacts from a family member. Pastors can be the most powerful community notable to whom ethnic families have access.

Educator

One role frequently assigned to the clergy is that of educator. In this context, the clergy can educate older persons not just in church-related matters but in ways that can enrich their lives generally. The clergy can also educate the non-elderly, both family members and others, as to better ways to relate to the elderly so that both the non-elderly and the elderly benefit.

For older Euro-Americans and those with whom they relate, this education can include an increased awareness of the cultural context of their homeland. The elderly themselves often lack the perspective to explain their behavior and the differences between their expectations and more contemporary U.S. expectations, but both the elderly and the family members have sufficient respect for members of the clergy to attend to what they say. Further, these clergy have the capacity to understand the changes in values, expectations, and day-to-day living situations experienced by the elderly Euro-Americans and to communicate this knowledge to others.

SOME CURRENT PROBLEMS

Forty years ago it was possible to say that the vast majority of churches were doing little for their members (Maves & Cedarleaf, 1949). Today this is no longer the case. All major denominations have issued formal statements on ministry to the elderly, and most have inaugurated programs for use by local congregations. Nonetheless, relatively few pastors have any specific preparation for working with older persons, and the need still far surpasses the available services.

In addition to the lack of gerontological training among pastors, there are other problems that inhibit services to these individuals. One is the rapid aging and high death rate of Euro-American immigrants. As long as a significant number still exist, there will continue to be some ethnically oriented services. When illness and death reduce that number, such services will no longer be available for the survivors and the newly aged.

A second concern is that the very success of Euro-Americans has paved the way for movement to suburban communities and relocation to other cities and towns where the individual cannot find clusters of his/her ethnic group. These population shifts increase possibilities of acculturation and assimilation, and they tend to isolate from their ethnic communities those Euro-Americans who are or soon will be elderly. Gentrification can accomplish the same end through a reverse process.

Also requiring attention is the aging of Roman Catholic religious and their decline in numbers, due largely to recruitment problems. The same is true among some Protestant denominations, but the causes lie more with reduced attendance and therefore fewer openings for young clergy. Older Euro-Americans will need to become accustomed to fewer young people in their congregations and more tasks performed by deacons and the laity.

CONCLUSION

The religious triad—faith, clergy, church—is pervasive in the lives of older Euro-Americans. Those individuals who are more acculturated or more assimilated may find it more difficult to comprehend the extent to which this triad is an intrinsic part of the daily lives of these persons. In this book, we have artificially separated religion/church from family and neighborhood, but in doing this we know we are looking at one piece that in actuality needs to be seen as part of the whole.

As we examine the role of the church and synagogue in relation to the elderly, we may propose an ideal congregation for our purposes: it has a high proportion of first-generation members; an ethnic-language-speaking, bilingual pastor; cultural organizations and celebrations in which the elderly are both participants and spectators; a committee composed in part of older people that function as advocate, program-planner, and general resource; and specialists in aging available for both direct services and to consult with the pastor.

Ironically, just as gerontological training of clergy and church/ synagogue staff is beginning to bear fruit, the ethnic neighborhood and the ethnic congregation seem to be offering a diminishing presence. Those who accept the importance of ethnically sensitive and gerontologically informed congregational response to the needs of the elderly must advocate effectively for such a priority in the face of the diminishing numbers of Euro-American elderly. Perhaps the growing frailty of many of these persons will lend credibility to that challenge to congregational leaders.

PART III:
Programs and Services

8

Ethnicity and Aging: Implications for Service Organizations

Zev Harel, Ph.D.

ETHNICITY, WELL-BEING, AND VULNERABILITY

Since the decade of the 1960s there has been a significant interest, theoretically and professionally, concerning the role of ethnicity in contemporary American life. Social and behavioral scientists studied the importance of ethnicity in determining cultural norms, political behavior, residential location, occupational status, educational aspirations, family structure, social integration, and informal care. Simultaneous with the growing interest reflected by scientific literature, there has been increased interest within the gerontological community concerning the role that ethnicity has in determining the well-being and service needs of the aged, including the availability of informal support in times of need.

It has been only more recently, however, that applied gerontological researchers and professionals in the fields of health and human services have begun to systematically pay attention to the ways in which ethnicity may impact on the lives of the ethnic elderly. For the purposes of this chapter the term *ethnicity* represents a group of people sharing the same identity as related to or influenced by cultural, religious, and/or language characteristics (Bonutti, 1974). Operationally, ethnicity includes elements of ethnic identification and affiliation as well as ethnic customs and practices. With the demographic changes in the U.S. population that have brought about an increase in the older age groups and a corresponding increase in demand and need for service (Harel, Wyatt, & Luick, 1984), the exploration of the importance of ethnicity for the well-being, vulnerability, and service needs of the aged becomes more crucial. As Marjorie Cantor (1976) states in her research:

> Meaningful social planning requires precise knowledge of both the extent to which the aging process is similar for all older people and the degree to which racial, ethnic, and socioeconomic differences require varying types of community facilities and services to sustain older people independently in the community for as long as possible. (p. 242)

Only after the function of ethnicity in the lives of the elderly has been better understood can health and human service professionals plan and organize more effective services for these elderly.

There are two ways in which ethnicity may impact on the well-being and/or vulnerability of the aged. On the one hand, it may function advantageously; persons with higher levels of integration into ethnic groups may be more inclined to practice self-reliance and engage in self-help and mutual-help efforts. These ethnic elderly may also have more extensive and meaningful informal social support networks. A higher level of ethnic connectedness is likely to contribute to the vitality, viability, and social integration of the neighborhood in which they live. Neighborhood integration, in turn, is likely to increase the availability of informal support and reduce the need for the reliance on public services. For the frail and impaired aged, it is likely to reduce the need for institutionalization and costly long-term care services.

On the other hand, membership in an ethnic community may work to the disadvantage of some adults and aged. Lack of acculturation to the contemporary ways of American life may inhibit or prevent the elderly from taking advantage of opportunities available in the community. Language, cultural, and residential barriers, as well as a cultural inhibition against asking for assistance, may isolate the ethnic elderly from available services. The function of these barriers in the lives of the ethnic elderly cannot be underestimated. Even the best-intentioned service can fail if these cultural factors are not adequately taken into consideration. To better understand the service needs of ethnic aged, research on the well-being and service needs of the ethnic aged and literature on service use among the aged are reviewed and discussed. A realistic understanding of vulnerability and service needs among elderly members of ethnic communities offers direction for more effective planning of service efforts that are required to assure the safety, security, and well-being of ethnic aged.

WELL-BEING AND SERVICE NEEDS AMONG ETHNIC AGED

There are two conflicting contentions in the professional literature regarding the use of ethnic variables in service use research. Holzberg (1982) contends that cultural variables are often ignored by researchers. White Americans, in her view, are generally placed in one category as long as they are of a similar socioeconomic status and background. Such an approach ignores many important factors that may be of critical importance in the planning of services. Markides (1982), however, asserts that researchers fail to produce sufficient evidence that ethnic–cultural factors as well as ethnic–minority status are of critical significance. In his view, this is mainly the reason that researchers tend not to include cultural and ethnicity variables in their conceptual formulations.

Perhaps because of this methodological dispute, the importance of ethnicity in determining the need for services and service utilization has received only marginal attention in gerontological literature. In general, the work that has been done to date is exploratory in nature (Eribes & Bradley-Rawls, 1978; Fandetti & Gelfand, 1976; Guttmann et al., 1979a; Kandel, 1979). There have been relatively few attempts to construct models that contain salient dimensions necessary for understanding service needs, use, and outcome among the ethnic elderly.

The necessity for more research that seeks to guide the development of models for the planning and organization of services to elderly members of various ethnic communities is indicated by the results from studies of Chinese aged. Recent research indicates that many previously accepted notions about Chinese-American life and culture are no longer valid. Chen (1979) disputes the contention that the Chinese elderly are at a cultural advantage because of the filial piety that characterizes traditional Chinese society. He asserts that because of the overwhelming presence of the American value system the elderly Chinese find themselves at a decided disadvantage when compared with their elderly White counterparts. Their culture is acting more as a hindrance than a help in confronting the problems of old age. An inability to speak English combines with other barriers and causes these elderly to restrict their associations to people who, like themselves, are disadvantaged by the circumstances of their lives. Fujii (1976) also disputes the notion that Asians take care of their elderly. Carp and Kataoka (1976) substantiate in their research the disadvantaged status of the Chinese aged. They found that Chinese aged are hindered by lack of knowledge and by negative attitudinal predispositions toward the use of Western medical services.

Another common misconception about the ethnic aged is that it is only the poor ethnic aged who are having difficulty adjusting to the cultural mainstream and are therefore unable or unwilling to make use of available services. Kandel (1979) found in her study of three ethnic groups in a large housing complex that each group tended to stratify itself into a separate and clearly distinct social group. Linn (1979) notes that in the case of the Cuban aged, problems are caused by uprootedness along with the other difficulties experienced by ethnic aged. Research has also shown that many ethnic elderly strive to maintain the ethnic content of their lives and the lives of their children, perhaps through language instruction or by pursuing hobbies of ethnic origin. This interest in their ethnic heritage can have very positive effects, but when it is impossible for the elderly to express their ethnicity in this manner, depression and alienation often occur (Mostwin, 1979). These circumstances may occur at any income level, not simply among the poor.

Knowledge about the importance of ethnicity is, therefore, not only interesting theoretically but of considerable importance for the planning and organization of health and social services. Many elderly who live in ethnic neighborhoods and/or are affiliated with ethnic institutions may have access to informal sources of support and to services they prefer, which, in the long run, may be less expensive than traditional means of providing services. Biegel and Sherman (1979) suggest that more use be made of the neighborhood and the ethnic community.

Research has indicated that the ethnic population does not tend to take advantage of health services (Biegel & Sherman, 1979;

Guttmann et al., 1979a). Kahana & Felton (1977) found in a Midwestern city that services were more readily available for Jewish, compared with Polish, aged. Guttmann et al. (1979a) found in their research that, in general, ethnic group members preferred to receive assistance from their own families. If that was not possible, their next source of preferred assistance was an ethnic or church-related organization. The reason for this is not only a lack of knowledge about the availability of resources but also an inhibition against leaving the ethnic community to make use of those resources. Merely locating the health services in the ethnic community does not necessarily solve these problems. Interviews with ethnic aged reveal an unwillingness to deal with people perceived as outsiders. Often, the reason for this is the inability to communicate in English.

Because they do not reach out for assistance, the ethnic elderly, especially those who were left behind by their culturally and geographically mobile children, frequently find themselves isolated, both physically and mentally. This isolation leads to a worsening of their condition. When help finally arrives it is often of the wrong kind. Markson (1979) has noted that the ethnic elderly are much more likely to be placed in mental institutions. Often this is done not on the basis of a diagnosed mental disturbance but because of the perceived difficulty of dealing with the ethnic aged and the erroneous perception that mental institutions provide cheaper care than alternative forms of health and human services.

Service providers have generally tended to ignore a potentially powerful tool for aiding the ethnic aged: the ethnic community. Before service professionals can make proper use of the community as a resource, more must be learned about the ethnic aged and their environment. It is not always possible to apply findings from one ethnic community to another. Guttmann et al. (1979a) discovered in their research that there was a great deal of variation between ethnic groups. Therefore, each group must be studied separately to determine the advantages and disadvantages of being an elderly member of a particular ethnic community. Giordano (1973) in his study of the effects of ethnicity on mental health among ethnic aged emphasizes the need for more research in this area and says that neighborhood-based research ought to be carried out along with broader studies. This would allow for the ethnic factor to be more adequately recognized and accepted.

Ethnic, cultural, and class distinctions can determine the patterns of certain illnesses and the use of services. Concern about ethnicity should be as automatic to researchers as investigations into the history and prevalence of illness and epidemiological studies are for doctors.

As Guttmann et al. (1979a) have stated, more systematic evidence is desirable concerning the status and service needs of elderly members of ethnic communities. Additionally, data on the interests, resources, and ability of ethnic communities to serve the needs of their elderly members are scarce. Future applied ethnic research should continue to focus on the health and functional status as well as social interaction and social integration patterns among ethnic aged. This research will provide a more systematic data base on the state of well-being and vulnerability of ethnic aged with regard to their health and social needs. It is also necessary to study factors that lead to withdrawal and social isolation among ethnic elderly. In this regard it is important to ascertain the effects of declining social activity and participation on the morale and mental health of the ethnic aged. This research will provide data on the mental health of the ethnic aged. There is also a necessity to investigate the perceived service needs and service utilization patterns of ethnic aged, including those of the unaffiliated and those who lack informal support.

More systematic data are necessary on the role and importance of ethnic communities in meeting the needs of ethnic aged. There is a need to ascertain the resources available in ethnic communities along with the expertise, capabilities, and willingness of those communities to serve as focal points in caring for their aged. There is an indication for the necessity study the potential role of ethnic organizations as sources of support and mediating structures for the elderly. There is also a need to study the ways in which ethnic communities may become focal points for meeting the psychological and mental health needs, the social activity, and spiritual needs of their elderly members.

Findings from such research not only would provide a better informational base on the well-being, vulnerability, and service needs of ethnic elderly, but also would highlight the resources available and the willingness and capabilities of ethnic communities to play various roles in meeting the service needs of ethnic aged.

SERVICE USE RESEARCH

To better understand the service needs of ethnic aged, it may be useful to review service needs, service use, and predictors of service use among the aged. In recent years interest has increased in the well-being and service needs of the older population. In part this interest is stimulated by the increase in demand for services by persons in older age groups. A growing effort is also being made to understand the importance of ethnic and racial differences as they affect disadvantaged status and service needs in the advanced years of life (Jackson & Harel, 1983).

As is evident from current population reports and gerontological research, the number of older persons in the United States has been steadily increasing and is projected to continue to rise. The highest growth rates are projected for the oldest age groups (Brotman, 1977). Age and impairment in health and functional status are highly associated. With increased age the prevalence of chronic illnesses and functional impairments also rises (Brody, 1977). Older persons are likely, therefore, to need and utilize health and social services in the community as well as in institutional settings. Service agencies in the field of aging have been providing care for older individuals and families who need home-based services as well as for those who need and are able to use the services available at nutrition sites and other agencies in the community.

The most prevalent need among the vulnerable aged is for long-term care services. This need is largely determined by decline in functional competence, impairment in mental functioning, and the incidence of chronic disease and disability. Elderly persons, by virtue of their high risk of functional and mental limitations and incidence of chronic disease and disability, are the primary recipients of long-term care services. Increased need and demand for long-term care services are brought about by the increase in the older U.S. population as a whole, and more important, by the fact that there has been a more rapid increase in the higher age groups. Since this aging pattern of the population is projected to continue until the year 2030, the number of persons at highest risk of functional impairment and high incidence of chronic disease, disability, and need of long-term care services will rise accordingly (Doty, Liu, & Wiener, 1985).

These population trends among the aging will continue to increase the demand for long-term care services in the future. Although nursing home care is the most visible form of long-term care, most of the disabled are cared for at home by friends and relatives. Long-term care is characterized by medical, personal, social, and psychological care over extended time periods. The need for long-term care is not necessarily identified with particular diagnoses but rather with a configuration of physical or mental disabilities and an impairment of the functions necessary for daily living.

Although such conditions affect individuals of all ages, the need for long-term care and assistance with activities of daily living greatly increases with age (Dunlop, 1980). Only 2.6% of persons aged 65 to 74 years require assistance with personal care compared with 31.6% of those 85 years of age and over. It is estimated that in the United States 8 million persons, two thirds of whom are elderly, need assistance with personal care (Brody, 1977).

While 29% of the long-term care population reside in an institutional setting (for example, nursing homes), 71% are in the community. Generally, residents of institutions are more disabled than dependent elderly in the community; yet for every person 65 years of age and over residing in a nursing home, there are more than twice as many persons living in the community and requiring similar levels of care.

Informal care, primarily by family, constitutes the bulk of care to the disabled elderly who require assistance in activities of daily living. Formal sources of care (paid providers of home health, homemaker/chore services, adult day-care programs, and so forth) provide a minority of the care to the disabled elderly. In 1982, formal services accounted for less than 15% of all *helper days of care* in the community (Comptroller General, 1977b; Dunlop, 1980; Harel, Luick, & Wyatt, 1983).

Research indicates that long-term care service consumers, compared with cross-sections of aged populations, are generally older, are predominantly female, and have more limited economic and social resources. Furthermore, those receiving home-based services are more impaired than those who utilize services in the community (Comptroller General, 1977b; Harel et al., 1984).

The less impaired elderly need and use nutritional services, socialization opportunities, preventive health services, chore services, information and referral, and other services that fulfill an important function in assuring them access to benefits and services that provide them with care and assistance. These services are offered in the community because of the realization that a sizable fraction of older persons needs care and assistance from service agencies.

With the recognition of the needs of the more impaired aged, consistent efforts have been made in recent years to better plan and target services to those aged who are most vulnerable and have the most limited economic and social resources. The Older Americans Act, implemented through State Offices on Aging and Area Agencies on Aging, has fostered attempts to assess service needs systematically and to develop comprehensive and coordinated services for older persons (Administration on Aging, 1979). Service utilization research indicates that, in addition to sociodemographic characteristics and health and functional status impairment, information about benefits and services play important roles in the prediction of service utilization (Krout, 1983; Silverstein, 1984). Not all older people are likely to have information about resources and services that might directly enhance the quality of their lives (Branch, 1978). A literature review by Silverstein (1984) reveals that lack of knowledge about resources and services is likely to reduce both the search for services and the search for information about services. Findings from empirical investigations reveal that some older persons do not know what benefits are available, nor to which ones they are entitled; others with medical problems do not know that there are agencies to which they could turn; and only a small fraction of widows were found to be familiar with the procedures used by service agencies (Katz, Gutch, Kahn, & Barton, 1975; Kent & Matson, 1972; Lopata, 1973).

Silverstein's review (1984) further indicates that even when people have a general knowledge about available services, they may not be able to relate them to their own needs or to the needs of others around them. Older persons may be unable to match their own needs with available services; they may not be inclined to use services, or they may not know how to negotiate services from service agencies (Bild and Havighurst, 1976; Cantor, 1976; Comptroller General, 1977b). In recent research on connected service users under the Older Americans Act, there was considerable variation found in knowledge about and access to services (Harel et al., 1984).

Powers and Bultena (1974) assert that distinctions need to be made between awareness of services, expressed intent to use services, and actual utilization of services. In a review of research on service use by the aged, Krout (1983) concludes that the perception of services among elderly, their access to services, and their intent to use services are far from uniform and/or consistent.

Along with knowledge, access, and attitudinal predisposition, informal support and the interface between formal and informal are also important determinants of service use among the elderly (Harél et al., 1983; Krout, 1983). The informal system is more likely to provide emotional support and assistance with personal care and household management. In contrast, the formal system of public and voluntary agencies provides entitlement to housing, education, safety, and transportation, as well as health and social services (Comptroller General, 1977b).

Data from empirical studies document that most older Americans have a viable and functioning informal support system, but that older persons and their informal caregivers turn to formal organizations for assistance when the nature of their problems becomes too difficult for them to handle alone (Cantor, 1976; Comptroller General, 1977b). One major survey of impaired elderly found that it was a spouse or adult child caregiver who helped with personal care tasks (Noelker & Poulshock, 1982). For the older population in general, 50% of all in-home services are provided by the family, and for those who are severely impaired, the rate climbs to 80% (Comptroller General, 1977b). Anderson, Patten, and Greenberg (1980) reported that 78% of home care service users received help from family and friends, and the informal system rendered significantly more care than did formal organizations.

The reviewed research reveals a growing need, demand, and use of community-based and institutional services. Research also indicates that in addition to objective states of health impairment and functional limitations, knowledge about benefits and services, access to services, and attitudinal predispositions toward the use of services play important roles in service utilization. Evidence indicates that informal sources of support have not only social and emotional value in assuring the security and well-being of older persons, but also an important role in reducing the need for and use of costly long-term care services. There has been little research to date, however, that ascertains the ways that membership in an ethnic group determines self-help, informal support, and knowledge about, access to, and attitudinal predisposition toward service utilization.

Guttmann et al. (1979a) assert that there are more than 40 million members of ethnic communities, constituting a sizable portion of our society, with approximately 4 million elderly among them. There is a need, therefore, for more systematic research that would ascertain the service needs and use of the elderly members of ethnic and minority groups and the ways that these groups may enhance the overall well-being of their aged members, especially the frail. In the absence of more systematic evidence, statements about the service needs of adult and aged members of ethnic communities are based on assumptions and, to a limited extent, on professional observations and research evidence. It appears reasonable to assert that ethnic aged may be characterized as having service needs similar to those identified for general cross-sections of aged populations. The vulnerable ethnic elderly need home-based and institution-based long-term care services. Members of their informal support system need assistance in coping with the burdens of caregiving. It may be assumed that the fraction of ethnic elderly residing in a family member's home or receiving extensive informal care may be somewhat higher than that found in cross sections of aged. Other elderly members of ethnic communities need access to benefits, resources, and services that will assure their safety, provide them with access to health and social services, and offer them opportunities for nutrition services, social interaction, and recreational opportunities. It may be assumed that religious, cultural, and spiritual needs of ethnic aged are likely to be more readily available in their respective communities.

VULNERABILITY AND SERVICE IMPLICATIONS

Along with the need for more systematic research, available data indicate that the ethnic elderly constitute a heterogeneous group with special needs, interests, and preferences. This recognition is essential for any serious attempt to plan interventions on their behalf. It appears appropriate, on the basis of the reviewed literature, to identify the ethnic elderly who should be of greatest concern to professionals and public officials in the fields of health and social services. Among the ethnic aged are those who have acculturated to the contemporary ways of American life, but a large number continue ethnic traditions and patterns of behavior. The literature does not clearly indicate, and therefore we may only hypothesize about, the ways in which ethnic connectedness and acculturation are interrelated and, in turn, affect well-being. It may be expected that ethnic adults and aged with higher levels of ethnic connectedness are more likely to engage in self-help and mutual help, have more extensive social support networks, and provide informal care. It may be further hypothesized that those with both higher levels of ethnic connectedness and higher levels of acculturation are likely to have the highest levels of overall well-being, to be contributors to mutual-help efforts, and to utilize more extensively resources and services made available through formal organizations.

Conversely, it may be expected that those ethnic aged with higher levels of ethnic connectedness and lower levels of acculturation will have less knowledge, less access, and more attitudinal predispositions that will preclude reliance on benefits and services. It may be expected, therefore, that aged with high ethnic connectedness and limited levels of acculturation who lack an informal support system may be the most vulnerable and most likely to have the most extensive degree of unmet service needs. The reviewed literature indicates the necessity to consider not only the service needs of the ethnic aged, along with the resources available within the ethnic communities to meet these needs, but also the extent to which the general service community engages in efforts to target services for ethnic aged.

There is a clear indication for the central importance of the informal support system, including children, family members, and friends, in the lives of ethnic elderly. Given a choice, a high percentage of ethnic aged would prefer to be aided in times of need by their family members. It is important to recognize, however, that the families of ethnic aged cannot shoulder all of the responsibility in meeting their service needs. In addition, there are a significant number of ethnic aged who do not have an adequate informal support system. Those without the benefit of a caring family would prefer to rely on friends and members of churches and ethnic groups in their respective communities. Even though there is no systematic evidence available, it may be hypothesized that elderly members of ethnic communities prefer to rely on members of their informal support system and on members of their ethnic communities to negotiate access to the formal service system when no other alternatives are available. In addition to the family, therefore, churches, other ethnic groups, and organizations need to be taken into consideration in efforts to meet the service needs of ethnic elderly.

In considering the service needs of ethnic elderly, it appears important to recognize that planning and practice efforts of health and human service professionals in the field of aging are guided by the following objectives: (a) to provide older individuals and families with effective services that are efficiently delivered; (b) to allow older service consumers as much discretion as possible in the services they use and enhance to the fullest extent possible their participation in the planning and provision of services; (c) to encourage and support family members, friends, neighbors, and volunteers in caring for older persons; and (d) to enhance the coping resources of older service consumers and their informal caregivers (Dunlop, 1980; Harel et al., 1985).

These service objectives are also appropriate for consideration in work with ethnic aged. Since service use research indicates that the search for and utilization of services is based to a considerable extent on knowledge about and access to services, as well as attitudinal factors, these must be of special concern in the planning and organization of services for elderly members of ethnic communities. There is a clear indication that service needs of the ethnic aged are to be considered, not only in the context of the resources available to meet these service needs within the ethnic communities but also in the extent to which the general service community engages in efforts to target services for ethnic aged.

Professional efforts to meet the service needs of the ethnic elderly are likely to be enhanced by the following activities:

- More effective dissemination of information about benefits and services available and to which all aged are entitled.
- Increased access on the part of the ethnic elderly to benefits and services.
- Creation of linking mechanisms between benefit offices, service agencies, and the ethnic elderly.
- Deliberate efforts to reduce attitudinal barriers and increase structural flexibility of benefit offices and service organizations.
- Concerted attempts to encourage mutual support and informal care, and to support the coping abilities of informal caregivers in ethnic communities.

- Special efforts to enhance the ability of ethnic groups and organizations to serve as mediators and service providers.
- Conscious attempts to meet the needs of the unaffiliated ethnic elderly and those who do not have the benefit of an informal support system.

Information Dissemination

Benefit offices, planners, and service providers need to engage in information dissemination activities directed toward elderly members of ethnic communities, members of their informal support system, and ethnic associations and organizations. They need to inform ethnic aged, members of their informal support system, leaders, and officers of ethnic organizations about the availability and accessibility of benefits and services. This may require innovative communication in the languages used by ethnic communities and also consideration of the unique preferences and communication style of ethnic communities.

There is a need for ongoing educational efforts to communicate about availability and application procedures related to benefits and services. This communication should be in the language used by members of the ethnic communities and may employ the services of newspapers, radio, and television. For the purposes of information dissemination, it is also important to employ the services of outreach workers, professionals, and paraprofessionals who are literate in the respective ethnic languages. Outreach dissemination efforts may be enhanced by enlisting the assistance of school children, young adults, and adult members of ethnic communities. Churches, synagogues, libraries, and ethnic organizations need to be seen as focal points for educational and dissemination activities.

Increasing Access

Educational and dissemination efforts are likely to improve the knowledge base of ethnic aged. To increase access to benefits and services, special outreach efforts are needed by service agencies to make contact with the ethnic elderly in their respective neighborhoods. It is essential to recognize the central importance, as shown by the data, of the informal support system for the ethnic elderly. Children, family members, and friends may serve as primary linking agents between the ethnic elderly and service organizations; family and other members of the informal support system must be considered in the planning of services. Additionally, churches, ethnic groups, and organizations often play a significant role in the lives of ethnic elderly. These ethnic institutions provide opportunities for involvement and affiliations, and they are sources of support for ethnic aged. Accessibility of services may be enhanced by locating satellite offices in ethnic neighborhoods; by recruiting elderly members of ethnic communities as volunteers and outreach workers; and by reliance on ethnic organizations, especially churches, synagogues, and senior groups for outreach efforts.

Attitudinal Predispositions

The utilization of benefits and services may be enhanced by a better understanding of attitudinal predispositions of ethnic elderly toward the use of services and a reduction of the stereotypical conceptions about ethnic elderly held by professionals. It is especially important to recognize that a sense of pride on the part of ethnic elderly may preclude their taking advantage of programs to which they are entitled. With proper outreach they may be informed that neighbors use such benefits and programs. Religious and ethnic leadership may also legitimize and encourage the use of benefits and services to which older persons may be entitled and thereby influence the attitudinal predisposition of the ethnic aged. These efforts may be enhanced by the employment of professionals with knowledge of ethnic communities and by the use of neighborhood-based satellite offices in religious institutions and civic organizations within ethnic communities.

Utilization of services is also affected by organizational characteristics. Stereotypical conceptions about ethnic aged in which they are depicted as either not needing or not wanting services may limit their use of services. Some older ethnic aged and members of their informal support system may have greater difficulty in penetrating the boundaries of bureaucratic health and social service organizations, especially those aged who have not acculturated to contemporary American life. They may also have greater difficulty with the fragmented service system, which requires consistent and active pursuit of benefits and services. The consideration of special ethnic preferences in food and the location of a nutrition site within the boundaries of the ethnic community may enhance the use of services offered through community-based service centers.

Service planners and service providers need to become better acquainted with the role and importance of social support networks in providing care and services for the ethnic elderly. When advising family members of the ethnic elderly, professionals need to be sensitive to the older persons' involvement and relationship in their network of informal social support. Practitioners should become aware of past and present relationships and interdependencies, and of the fact that ethnic elderly may resist the use of services until these are sanctioned and/or reinforced by members of their informal support system and by leaders of their churches and ethnic organizations. Respect and understanding for the needs and preferences of service consumers, coupled with effective communications with the elderly and members of their informal support system, are essential in work with all aged. A thorough understanding of ethnic and cultural factors, and the role of the ethnic social support system is critical if service providers are to plan adequately for the service needs of ethnic elderly.

Education, communication, and outreach efforts with members of the ethnic elderly's informal support system and with the informal leadership of the ethnic community may also be instrumental in reducing organizational barriers for the ethnic aged. Because ethnic elderly may not trust outsiders, they may not follow the directives of service providers and therefore resist the use of services. Resistance, in turn, may be misinterpreted by professionals who have not considered the influence of cultural factors. The result may be failure in communication efforts with ethnic elderly.

Encouraging Informal Support

Evidence indicates that the families of the ethnic elderly provide them with much attention and assistance in times of need. Family members, friends, and neighbors should be seen as important resources that require community and professional support. It is necessary to recognize that care of impaired elderly is associated with a considerable burden, that the family of ethnic aged cannot meet all of the service-related needs of the elderly, and that the coping skills and resources of informal caregivers themselves require support. Some relief and assistance for caregivers may be accomplished through the establishment of mutual-help networks and through providing informal caregivers' information about community resources. We must improve ways to reinforce neighborhood and mutual support groups among informal caregivers. Service planners need to work more directly with leaders of ethnic communities in planning services. Also, service providers need to work directly with the ethnic aged and with members of their support system in responding to their service needs.

Neighborhood and Ethnic Organizations

It is important to realize that most Euro-American elderly have various degrees of affiliation with churches, ethnic groups, and other organizations. In addition, ethnic communities have restaurants, food stores, and other conventional services frequented by ethnic elderly. The importance of these organizations should be recognized both as focal points for the delivery of services and as mediating structures between the ethnic elderly and the formal system of benefits and services. Some neighborhoods have self-help groups. These should be encouraged to address the needs of the elderly. In this context, it should be noted that there has been an increase in the emphasis to shift responsibility for service delivery from the national level, through the state and counties, to the local communities. The local communities and neighborhoods are better able to identify and represent the needs of their members. Advocacy on behalf of the needs of ethnic elderly may be undertaken by individual ethnic communities and also by coalitions of ethnic communities.

Planning for the Needs of the Unaffiliated

It is important to recognize that there are a significant number of ethnic aged who do not have an adequate support system; others may not be affiliated with ethnic groups and organizations. Since services are not readily available in the community, unaffiliated and unacculturated ethnic aged may find themselves in especially difficult situations. Ethnic elderly without an adequate informal support system may have difficulty getting the services they need. Because many ethnic groups do not have the expertise and the resources to plan and offer services, the unaffiliated ethnic elderly need to be of special concern to planners and service providers. Homebound and institutionalized ethnic elderly who lack adequate informal support should be of special concern to planners and service providers.

CONCLUSION

Concerns about the well-being, vulnerability, and service needs of Euro-American elderly need to be seen as an integral part of organized efforts to assure the safety, security, and well-being of all aged. Efforts need to be directed to assure that policies, legislative enactments, and programs will encourage the targeting of services to benefit those elderly who are in greatest need. Planning and service agencies need to consider the special needs of Euro-American aged along with the resources of their ethnic communities. Respect and understanding of the needs and preferences of service consumers, coupled with effective communication with the elderly and members of their informal support system, are essential in work with all aged, but are particularly important in work with ethnic elderly. Finally, advocacy efforts must be continued on the local, state, and national levels in cooperation with the leadership of the ethnic communities to assure progress in meeting the service needs and providing for the well-being of all aged, including those who are members of ethnic communities.

9

The Role of Government in Providing Support for the Euro-American Elderly

*Christopher L. Hayes, Ph.D.,
and James J. Burr, M.S.W.*

In 1979 at a symposium on Euro-American elderly held at The Catholic University of America, the former Assistant Secretary for Neighborhood Development of the Department of Housing and Urban Development, the late Monsignor Geno Baroni, noted that "Americans are the most racially, culturally, ethnically, and regionally different people in the world; and there must be tolerance for diversity because it's a key to our survival." Besides advocating that our society must continue to recognize and respect this cultural diversity, Baroni encouraged the fostering of a partnership between the public and private sector in developing programs for the ethnic elderly. To give meaning to Baroni's vision, attention needs to be given to what role government should play in responding to the needs of the Euro-American elderly and how the private sector can make government more responsive in addressing social service concerns.

For purposes of this discussion, we are defining government in a broad sense that encompasses federal, state, and local entities that are mandated to deliver fiscal, planning, and coordinative functions on behalf of the elderly. At the federal level this would include the Administration on Aging of the Department of Health and Human Services, the Federal Council on Aging, and the Civil

Rights Commission; at the state level, the state units on aging; and in local government, the Area Agencies on Aging and city departments for the aged. In particular, we need to analyze how these government units have historically responded to the unique needs of the Euro-American elderly and what future efforts can be brought to bear by various groups to advocate for the needs of their older ethnic adults. One important role of these governmental entities is to establish for our nation's elderly social policies that address a variety of age-related concerns.

A major concern is how these governmental bodies will respond to the development of policy that assists the Euro-American elderly. The reality of today is that enacting social policies to address particular needs involves a highly politicized process that includes advocacy, special interest groups, lobbying, and money— all leading toward influence with elected and appointed officials (Torres-Gil, 1983). It is fair to say that European groups have yet to plunge into the political process to forge policies that respond to the needs of their elderly members. Reasons for this will be explored later, but it is important to note that the increase of advocacy organizations for the minority elderly have important implications for any political/advocacy efforts developed on behalf of the Euro-American elderly. Thus, the experience gained by different minority groups both to advocate for and to receive resources from the bureaucratic/political system will be integrated into this chapter.

A BRIEF HISTORICAL PERSPECTIVE

In determining what should be government's role in assisting the Euro-American elderly, it is critical that we review various factors that have influenced and continue to dominate governmental policies relating to ethnic immigrant groups in America. During the 1960s, public policy development made two radical shifts in addressing ethnic/minority groups that were obviously not melting into the American mainstream. Becoming more sensitive to individual group differences, the federal government reviewed the status of various minorities in America and concluded that direct federal involvement was necessary if assimilation was ever to be fully achieved.

Identifying racism and poverty as the root of the minority problem, the federal government developed actions that would make minorities indistinguishable from the general population as the first step in the assimilation process. To institute the amalgamation process of these minorities, the Great Society programs were instituted and culminated in the creation of the Office of Economic Opportunity in 1964 and the Demonstration Cities and Metropolitan Act of 1966. Each of these programs attempted to amalgamate minorities through greater economic and educational opportunities, improved housing, and more efficient social delivery systems.

The overall effect was to provide real opportunities for upward mobility for Blacks, Hispanics, and other minorities from central and eastern Europe, the Near East, and Asia, who had come to America following the repression in the Eastern Bloc during the 1950s.

The second ethnic phenomenon that occurred in the 1960s came to be identified as the *new pluralism,* which was a radical departure from the melting pot orientation. In the beginning, it was essentially cultural in focus and concentrated on the need of ethnic minorities to achieve a sense of legitimacy for their ethnic diversity. The new pluralists were not interested in assimilation or amalgamation. On the contrary, their major concern was with the perpetuation of their unique heritage. As the 1960s came to an end, certain other ethnic groups, following the lead of the visible minorities, began to demand a greater sensitivity and responsiveness from the federal government.

An important milestone for ethnic Americans, and the single most important accomplishment of the new pluralists during the beginning of their activity, was the passage of the Ethnic Heritage Studies Act of 1971, which provided, for the first time in our history, a federally funded program for the preservation and development of America's rich ethnic diversity and gave legitimacy to the positive, constructive force it could have in our society. This act was perceived by many ethnic leaders as an event that signaled the demise of the melting pot as an American societal ideal. Cultural pluralism, they concluded, was now to be the standard for social policy development within the federal establishment. Many predicted that the 1970s would go down in American history as the Decade of the Ethnic.

Unfortunately, the 1970s never lived up to pluralist expectations. Testifying before the U.S. Civil Rights Commission, Dr.

Myron B. Kuropas, former Special Assistant to the President for Ethnic Affairs in the Ford administration, characterized the 1970s for ethnic Americans:

> Some American ethnic groups have watched their lovingly preserved neigh-
> borhood destroyed by ill-conceived and poorly administered government
> housing programs. They have been forced to permit the busing of their
> children to schools located in communities that really didn't want them.
> Supreme Court decisions notwithstanding, they still believe affirmative-action
> programs are really a form of reverse discrimination which penalizes those
> who are least able to absorb the socio-economic penalty. And yet, despite two
> decades of efforts to sensitize the Federal bureaucracy to the values of the
> pluralistic model, their pleas to their Government are either politely ignored
> or dismissed as racist in origin (U.S. Civil Rights Commission, 1979).

Today, ethnic Americans on the whole continue to believe that the federal government is insensitive to their dual heritage and needs. In fact, the issue of one's dual heritage has recently created a problem within government circles. Writing in the 1981 summer issue of *Foreign Affairs,* Senator Charles McC. Mathias (R-MD) was critical of "ethnic groups which sometimes press causes that derogate from the national interest" (p. 977). For Mathias the question of dual loyalty is an important consideration in assessing the recent efforts of Jews, Irish, Greeks, and eastern European groups to influence American foreign policy initiatives. In many instances, argues Mathias, the pressures of these groups have led to policies that were ultimately counterproductive and in some cases even harmful to American interests. "Ethnicity enriches our life and culture and for that purpose should be valued and preserved," concludes Mathias, "but the problems of the modern world and their solution have broken past the boundaries of ethnic group, race, and nation" (p. 998).

A singular effect of the dual heritage in the Irish group, for example, is the result of the financial support provided to the Irish Republican Army by some Irish Americans, with the resulting devastation to the people in Northern Ireland.

Although progress can be seen in the acceptance of Euro-American diversity, the federal government has yet to recognize fully its legitimacy. As Kolm (1980) notes:

> Two centuries of assimilationist and melting pot indoctrination have in-
> timidated Euro-Americans and undermined their belief in the legitimacy and
> value of their ethnic patterns to society and even to their children, and

consequently, their self-confidence has been weakened. Their traditional defense against societal pressures and prejudice remains withdrawal to their own communities. As a result, some of the Euro-American groups never joined the mainstream of society and do not feel part of the American Society (p. 6).

GOVERNMENT ADDRESSING EURO-AMERICAN CONCERNS

From the above, it is not difficult to understand why many Euro-American elderly are both cautious and suspicious of many government-sponsored programs that would address their needs. However, other factors also affect how those of Euro-American backgrounds view government. Especially among earlier arriving European immigrants there is a strong self-reliant tradition that negates any desire for the government to provide aid. More recent European refugees who are fleeing the tyranny of totalitarian regimes tend to view all government with defiance and distrust.

As indicated in previous chapters, the Euro-American elderly as a group underutilize available services, benefits, and programs. Although a high percentage of Euro-American elderly would prefer to utilize family, friends, or church members in times of crisis, evidence exists that language and cultural barriers prevent the use of various governmental programs and services (Guttmann et al., 1979a). In addition, many Euro-American elderly are too proud to receive such assistance and are excluded from participation due to bureaucratic red tape, inflexible rules, and culturally insensitive personnel. To what extent should government be involved in addressing the cultural/linguistic needs of these elderly and reducing barriers to participation in services and benefits?

Two opposing positions can be identified in regard to federal government intervention in assisting the Euro-American elderly. One perspective believes that the European immigrant has had more than enough opportunities to master English, and any federal initiative to assist them to access public programs and benefits would be too costly. Furthermore, the wide diversity of languages and cultures that are encompassed under the Euro-American umbrella makes practical strategies unrealistic. Also, with the recent movement away from federal involvement in human service initiatives and more responsibility being placed on the private/local sector, no federal government intervention is warranted.

Those in favor of greater federal involvement on behalf of the Euro-American elderly argue that developing public policy that would strengthen local institutions such as the family, the neighborhood, the church, and the voluntary organization would greatly assist the Euro-American elderly. To counter the assumption that these immigrants did not want to learn English, arguments are made that because of their poor socioeconomic status upon arrival, they had to go to work immediately and could not avail themselves of free educational opportunities. Thus, government intervention at this time is both warranted and needed.

Within the last 10 years the federal government has, to some extent, recognized the plight of the Euro-American elderly. For example, the 1978 President's Commission on Mental Health found that many minority elderly (including Euro-American elderly) are not receiving appropriate services even though social, economic, and environmental factors render them particularly vulnerable to physical, psychological, and emotional problems. An important finding of the commission was that many government-funded or -operated programs often ignore existing cultural, social, and community supports. The above issues were also reflected in the 1979 U.S. Civil Rights Commission hearings, which outlined the various problems and concerns of Euro-American groups in the United States. Next, the 1981 White House Mini-Conference on Euro-American Elderly, held in Baltimore and Cleveland, provided an opportunity for representatives from government and ethnic circles to engage in a dialogue regarding concerns of the aging.

THE WHITE HOUSE MINI-CONFERENCES ON EURO-AMERICAN ELDERLY

The two White House Mini-Conferences on Euro-American elderly held in 1980 and 1981 were a clear recognition on the part of the federal government of the Euro-Americans as a new entity among the minorities within the elderly population. Representatives of the Euro-American elderly were very firm and vocal in their contention that the needs of the so-called White ethnic elderly must be translated into action programs that would do justice to these people. Of particular importance was the emphasis on the role of the mediating structures in enhancing well-being in old age. Ethnic leaders and professional service providers echoed the wishes of elderly Euro-Americans by making the following recommendations:

- The federal government should regulate its own bureaucracy by requiring its agencies to submit an *ethnic impact statement* with each new change of personnel, programs, or procedures.
- The federal government should require that every governmental advisory council reflect in its membership the ethnic and age composition of the people served by the program.
- There should be more officials and administrators in the federal government who are sensitive to and supportive of the needs and interests of the Euro-American elderly, and these persons should be persons of Euro-American descent themselves.
- Funding should be designated for the translation and printing of information in a variety of ethnic languages on existing public benefits (Medicare, Medicaid, and so forth) to encourage the use of these support systems by the elderly who are members of various ethnic groups.
- Government should encourage the maintenance of ethnic identity in subsidized housing, nursing homes, and homes for the aged.

Because of space limitations we are unable to include the other recommendations made concerning government's role in enhancing mediating structures and neighborhoods, and in strengthening family life. However, three major themes concerning government's role can be gleaned from all of the recommendations made: (a) public policy must take into account the unique, distinct, culturally defined patterns of behavior of the Euro-American elderly, and relevant services must be oriented to their needs; (b) government must find strategies to strengthen the family, the ethnic neighborhood, and the church that act as critical supports to the Euro-American elderly in times of crisis; (c) government must develop and foster cooperative efforts between the public and voluntary sectors of society to ensure the economic, social, and physical well-being of the Euro-American elderly.

THE OLDER AMERICANS ACT AMENDMENTS OF 1982–1983

A variety of recommendations from the 1981 Mini-Conference were adopted in the Older Americans Act:

- Section 307 of the act provided for service workers fluent in the language spoken by a predominant number of older individuals to be employed in locations where substantial numbers of those older individuals reside. These service workers would assist the elderly who have language difficulties to learn what services were available and how to access them.
- Section 422 of the Older Americans Act encourages demonstration projects emphasizing the needs of low-income elderly persons who have limited English-speaking ability.
- Section 502 of the Act encourages states to make certain, through agreements with service providers, that the needs of limited-English-speaking, eligible individuals are taken into account in the development of projects under Title V of the act.

The intent of these amendments in the Older Americans Act was to ensure that organizations that receive Older Americans Act funds attempt to serve all of the older population. As an example, Section 705 of the original Title VII Older Americans Act nutrition program, which gave some attention to the ethnic elderly, reads, "that preference shall be given to projects serving low-income individuals and provide assurance that grants will be awarded to projects operated by and serving the needs of minority, Indian, and limited English-speaking eligible individuals in proportion to their number in the State" (U.S. Congress, 92nd Cong., P.L. 92-258). Unfortunately, as Bechill (1979) points out, the Administration on Aging has done little to address limited English-speaking elderly within Title VII nutrition programs to this date.

To our best understanding, the Administration on Aging has made few attempts to implement monitoring procedures that evaluate compliance of Sections 307, 422, and 502 of the Older Americans Act. An obvious vehicle to ensure compliance is to have the Administration on Aging, through its regional offices, mandate states to establish such monitoring procedures. In addition, attempts should be made to determine how many service workers, fluent in a European language, have been hired by states and Area Agencies on Aging to assist elderly Euro-American to obtain needed services and benefits.

It is our contention that the minimal role the federal government has played to date in assisting the Euro-American elderly with language difficulties could be greatly expanded. Historically, the Administration on Aging has made major attempts to ensure participation of the aged of low-income and minority groups in various programs under the Older Americans Act, particularly the Title III state and community service programs and the Title VII nutrition program (Bechill, 1979). This attention has been due largely to the commitment of Dr. Arthur S. Flemming, former U.S. Commissioner on Aging. From 1973 to 1978 major initiatives were directed toward the minority aged, defined as Black, Spanish-speaking, Asian-American, or Native American. Because the Euro-American had not been designated a "minority" group, similar attention to the needs of their elderly was not considered. However, the means by which various minority groups have received attention from the Administration on Aging and governmental agencies are worth reviewing for potential similar efforts to be instituted by various Euro-American groups.

ADVOCATING FOR ETHNIC/MINORITY ELDERLY

During the last decade advocacy by both the elderly themselves and national aging organizations has played a critical role in influencing the legislative process and increasing services for the aged. According to Stanford (1978), advocacy means "applying pressure to change the way in which services are delivered and insisting that services provided are reasonable in the environment in which the elders reside" (p. 129). It is clear that if Euro-American elders are to receive needed services, increased advocacy efforts on their behalf must occur. At the same time, specific attempts must be made to involve the Euro-American elderly in advocating on their own behalf. The recent formation of national minority aging organizations serve as an excellent example of the catalyst needed to engage the Euro-American elderly and ethnic organizations in advocating for increased access to existing service delivery systems.

Before 1971 advocates for minority aging concerns were unorganized and lacked both visibility and influence in the formulation of national policies on aging (Torres-Gil, 1983). The 1971 White House Mini-Conference on Aging played a strategic role in getting minority groups to recognize that their underrepresentation at the actual conference deserved increased advocacy on their part. Pressure exerted by Blacks, Hispanics, Asians, and Native Americans led to support by the Administration on Aging of the development of the following coalition of national aging organizations: the National Caucus on Black Aged, the National Hispanic Council on Aging, the Asociación Nacional Pro Personas Mayores, the National Indian Council on Aging, and the Pacific/Asian Resource Center on Aging. Each of these minority aging organizations has been instrumental in conducting research on the needs of their elderly, increasing the number of minorities on governmental peer review panels, influencing the development of legislation and regulations affecting minorities, and generally representing the needs of the minority elderly.

There is now no reason for the federal government to recognize a national coalition of Euro-American elderly, as it does Hispanic or Black minority groups. Why? Because there is no national coalition of the different ethnic groups representing varied European cultures. There is at present no consensus among them that spells out national goals and priorities for achieving such goals. As a matter of fact, current interethnic conflicts impede progress toward a national coalition. Therefore, recognition of a Euro-American elderly minority by the federal government must await a resolution of these difficulties.

It cannot be disputed that in a relatively short time these national minority aging organizations have encouraged the Administration on Aging to address each of their specific and unique needs. Unfortunately, the 1981 White House Mini-Conference on Euro-American Elderly did not result in a national coalition. At this time, five questions need to be addressed:

1. Why have Euro-American groups had difficulty in joining together to advocate for specific social concerns?
2. What is the role, if any, of the federal government in providing support to the Euro-American elderly?
3. Can the Administration on Aging be pressured to address the needs of the Euro-American elderly without the development of a national coalition?
4. Is there support for such a coalition among ethnic leaders?
5. What are the appropriate steps needed to form such a body?

PROBLEMS IN EURO-AMERICAN COALITION BUILDING

Conflict among different Euro-American groups was a regular part of American urban life throughout the early periods of immigration; and although this receives little political attention today, it still occurs. Glazer (1971) identifies three types of conflict that have developed between Euro-American groups: (a) ethnic succession—conflicts over potential control, specific values affected by public action, and jobs; (b) contrasting cultures—conflicts over different languages, behavior, religion, and life-styles; (c) federal government involvement—conflicts over the perception that one group is getting more assistance than another. These interethnic conflicts have played a critical role in the inability of these groups to form coalitions on a variety of social issues.

To understand this intergroup conflict, one must recognize that each Euro-American group, though similar in valuing strong family ties, respect for authority, and so on, is quite diverse. For example, Polish and Italian communities may share much in common, but their occupational history, patterns of influence, and relation to the Catholic Church are quite different.

How can these Euro-American groups be persuaded to come together? Who will enable and encourage them to recognize their mutual problems? The catalyst may well be the issue of the burgeoning elderly population if the issue can be articulated and organized.

Based on the previous experience of different minority groups, it is dubious whether the Administration on Aging would develop specific social policy initiatives for the Euro-American elderly without being pressured to do so by a unified ethnic-American special interest group. As mentioned earlier, the development of social policy is a highly politicized process requiring concerted advocacy efforts by a coalition. By definition, a coalition is an organization of diverse groups that combine their human and material resources to effect a specific change that the members are unable to bring about independently (Brown, 1984).

DEVELOPMENT OF A EURO-AMERICAN ELDERLY COALITION

The foundation of constituency-building is formulating an individualized strategy, not only for attracting a particular organization to the coalition but for assuring its long-range commitment (Brown, 1984). National leaders from different Euro-American communities might implement the following strategy toward developing an aging coalition:

- Develop an aging coalition composed of as many Euro-American groups as possible. Share unique contributions that each group can make and subordinate individual differences in order to facilitate a group effort.
- Define the specific social policies for the Euro-American elderly that need immediate attention. Publicize both the formation of the coalition and the desired social policies by enlisting all of the media, especially the ethnic media.
- Utilize ethnic gerontologists or those sympathetic to the needs of ethnic groups both to staff the coalition and to coordinate the solicitation of support from all aging organizations.
- Approach both the federal executive department and the U.S. Congress regarding the issues. Follow up meetings with letters to key decision-makers.
- Identify significant Americans of European origin who are recognized for their contributions to this country. Utilize birthday and anniversary celebrations as a means of continually seeking support from the American public. Develop petitions as a vehicle to convince Congress to give priority to this effort.
- Confirm in writing any federal government commitment to act on meeting the stated goals of the coalition. Seek and secure an exact timetable for federal government action.
- Monitor federal government efforts from their origin to their conclusion and assure that the action is institutionalized.

FEDERAL GOVERNMENT RESPONSES TO A EURO-AMERICAN ELDERLY COALITION

How would the federal government respond to such a coalition? It would seem that the Administration on Aging could take a variety of positive steps to satisfy the concerns of such a coalition. First, recognizing the need to support efforts that would advocate for both public and private cooperative efforts in addressing the needs of Euro-American elderly, the Administration on Aging could conceivably provide discretionary funding for the continued development of a national coalition. Such funding could enhance the possibility of fostering voluntary self-help efforts within ethnic neighborhoods that would not require additional government funds. In addition, funding such a coalition to expand gerontological training within ethnic organizations, senior services, and churches would ensure both appropriate use of existing aging resources and sensitivity to culturally appropriate interventions.

Second, the Administration on Aging could coordinate among other divisions of the Department of Health and Human Services the appropriate translation of government-sponsored programs into different Euro-American languages. For example, programs such as Social Security and Medicare, which are administered through Health and Human Services, could be guided by the Administration on Aging to produce documents in Euro-American languages. Similar efforts to translate pertinent information could be implemented by individual states and counties that administer Medicaid and Public Assistance (Income Maintenance for the Poor) and often have untranslated laws, regulations, and procedures.

Third, various efforts could be made to work with each regional Health and Human Services Office for Civil Rights to develop strategies to ensure that Euro-American elderly seeking health benefits are not the victims of discrimination due to national origin. Title 45 Code of Federal Regulations, Part 80, issued pursuant to Title VI of the Civil Rights Act of 1964, prohibits all health care providers who receive federal financial assistance from Health and Human Services from conducting any of their programs, activities, or services in a manner that subjects any person or class of persons to discrimination on the grounds of race, color, or national origin. A frequent cause of discrimination on the basis of national origin in health care settings that often leads to a violation of the Title VI regulation is the use of ineffective methods of communication between English-speaking health care providers and persons who, because of their national origin, have limited proficiency in using English (U.S. Dept. HHS, Office for Civil Rights, 1985).

THE ROLE OF STATE AND LOCAL GOVERNMENTS

Both state and local government entities play a pivotal role in coordinating and overseeing the funds granted through the Older Americans Act. Each state has a State Unit on Aging designated to develop and administer the state plan of the Older Americans Act and to be a focal point on aging in that state. On the local level, the Area Agency on Aging is designated by the state agency to develop and administer the area plan for a comprehensive and coordinated system of services for older persons. Since Congress amended the Older Americans Act in 1978, concern has mounted that minority and ethnic elderly have not had the opportunity to assist in the planning and implementation of programs under the Older Americans Act. This has resulted in the ethnic/minority elderly's not receiving adequate services, information, or assistance from the programs mandated by the Older Americans Act (U.S. Civil Rights Commission, 1982).

In planning services at the local level for the disbursement of Older Americans Act funds, the Area Agency on Aging must develop a 3-year service plan to submit to the State Unit on Aging for approval. This 3-year plan is to be reviewed through public hearings to evaluate whether the objectives and resulting programs address local aging concerns. A serious issue is whether various Euro-American leaders and elderly actually participate in such hearings. The 1985 National Conference on Euro-American Elderly disclosed that many ethnic groups and organizations are often unaware that such hearings are taking place or do not understand the planning process of the Older Americans Act. According to Estes (1979), participation of the elderly in public hearings, state plan reviews, and comment procedures under the Older Americans Act is minimal and symbolic.

Local Area Agencies on Aging that contain large numbers of Euro-American elderly within their jurisdiction have responsibility for the following:

1. Inform local ethnic organizations of public hearings concerning the disbursement of Older Americans Act funds through publicizing such activities within the ethnic media, specific mailings, and the like.
2. Translate public hearing notices in various Euro-American languages to attempt to gain ethnic elderly input.
3. Provide translators at such hearings to ensure that concerns are voiced.
4. Develop opportunities for Euro-American communities to understand the planning process mandated under the Older Americans Act.

Similarly, state plans submitted to the Administration on Aging should reflect both input from Euro-American elders and service strategies to address their needs. Such input is critical in light of the finding that state unit planning made very little use of outside input (Applied Management Sciences, 1975). In 1981 the Senate introduced an amendment to the Older Americans Act requiring specific state programs for geographically concentrated groups of non-English-speaking elderly. This amendment was to provide a full-time Administration on Aging employee to provide counseling, information, referral, and translation services to non-English-speaking older persons. This staff member would also have the responsibility of ensuring that local service providers are "aware of cultural sensitivities and . . . take into account linguistic and cultural differences " (Section 307 [a][17], Older Americans Act, 1965). To the best of our knowledge, little has been done to mandate the hiring of such employees.

The various ethnic groups representing Euro-Americans at the local and state levels should take upon themselves the responsibility of seeing that the 1981 amendment to the Older Americans Act requiring specific state programs for geographically concentrated groups is implemented in each state. It could take the form of establishing a state-level ombudsman for ethnic minorities, particularly elderly Euro-Americans and others, to see that the existing provisions of the Older Americans Act are carried out at the state and local (Area Agency) levels, with particular attention to those responsibilities listed above for Area Agencies on Aging.

An important way in which local government can help the Euro-American elderly is by lobbying at other levels of government for changes that can help them. For example, if a federally funded health clinic does not provide adequate translation assistance, local government can informally lobby for staff changes or sue on behalf of limited-English-speaking clients (although such suits are rare).

However, before local governments can lobby other governments at state and federal levels, they must first be lobbied themselves. The city and county political structures must be influenced to support the goals for elderly Euro-Americans of all ethnic or cultural origins and thus help the elderly to secure entitlements that are their right as citizens.

Single-issue politics, which this effort represents, can succeed only if those behind the movement can work together and submerge their cultural or other antipathies in the interest of the elderly, the common bond of them all.

The very nature of cultural pluralism argues against concerted action by divergent cultural groups. Thus, the issue must transcend local parochial, ethnic affinities and focus on the greater good—helping the elderly of all ethnic groups to participate in the rewards of citizenship.

The local city and county governments must be understood in their administrative as well as political context. If we do not know how they work, then we cannot influence them. An understanding of the administrative process as well as the political process is necessary. It is not enough to be familiar with key legislators in city, county, or state governments. Each government bureaucracy depends on a key staff of legislative or other committees of each entity, and the influence of these staff people is very pervasive. They should be known and should be courted as much for their knowledge and expertise as for their influence within the structure of their own government entity.

Some of the common denominators of the political process at city, county, and state levels are worthy of attention:

- Recognition of the power structure of city, county, and state governments is a must for those who would influence the legislative process at these levels.
- Any ethnic group must have a knowledgable and articulate spokesman when they approach city, county, and state legislators. Women leaders are equally as successful as men.
- Politicians in city, county, and state governments are influenced by large numbers of voters who can do them good or do them harm. A consensus of ethnic group leadership representing large numbers who are prepared to speak for all elderly Euro-Americans is the best way to influence politicians at any level of government.
- Leaders of the Euro-American elderly must be willing to spend time and money, when necessary, to influence city, county, or state governments to support the goals that have been set to help elderly Euro-Americans.
- It is evident but not always appreciated that the professional staff of city, county, or state governments can be very helpful to any group that tries to influence governments. Their help should be enlisted whenever possible.
- Because of the fact that many groups attempt to influence city, county, or state legislators on behalf of children, the elderly, the disabled, and other minorities, the use of mass communication is necessary. Publicity about the cause and the use of various techniques will secure the legislators' attention.

Demonstrations are more effective than brochures. Human interest topics are more effective than a three-person committee visit to a legislator.
- Politics is the art of the possible. Therefore, have original positions and fall-back positions.
- At every government level cultivate key politicians who are members of an ethnic group themselves.

CONCLUSION

Historically, government at the federal, state, and local levels has done little to recognize the unique cultural and linguistic needs of the Euro-American, and in particular, the elderly within these groups. Although there is a growing body of legislation targeted at limited-English-speaking elderly, government has not enforced or guided programs that would ensure that such needs are met. It is becoming increasingly clear that pressure needs to be exerted on both federal and local governments to respond to the concerns of Euro-American elderly. The vehicle to exert such pressure may be the development of a national Euro-American elderly coalition. Different minority groups have gained recognition for their concerns by advocating for needed legislation and receiving support from the Administration on Aging through the utilization of national coalitions.

10

Resources and Services Benefiting the Euro-American Elderly

Christopher L. Hayes, Ph.D.

It is evident that a variety of deficiencies exist within our aging network in addressing the social service needs of the Euro-American elderly. Many advocates of the Euro-American elderly believe that only through government funding can we mobilize the resources needed to address housing, nutrition, health, and other human needs. During the last several decades we have interpreted resources to mean monetary grants to fund social service programs, especially from the federal government. However, any strategy that depends solely on government funding to develop programs is doomed to fail in this era of fiscal constraint. A basic contention of this chapter is that ethnic communities have a number of untapped, nongovernmental resources that can be utilized in assisting the Euro-American elderly.

As mentioned in Chapter 6, ethnic communities have provided assistance historically to those immigrants seeking employment, food, health insurance, and so forth. Such resources continue to exist in ethnic communities and can be directed toward the elderly. Within the last decade certain ethnic communities have made great strides in identifying both governmental and nongovernmental resources to develop programs for the Euro-American elderly. If such resources and programs can be identified, further attempts can be made by ethnic communities to ensure the well-being of their older population.

The purpose of this chapter is threefold: (a) to identify resources in the ethnic community that can strengthen the heritage, traditions, and capabilities of the Euro-American elderly to care for themselves; (b) to describe innovative programs that can be replicated to meet the concerns of the ethnic aged in need of services; and (c) to describe public resources that can be utilized in concert with assistance generated from the ethnic community to strengthen community efforts in the provision of care for the Euro-American elderly.

Today, ethnic communities still contain religious, fraternal, and social welfare institutions that provide monetary contributions, volunteers, and programs to benefit different age groups. Besides these critical resources, ethnic communities contain private foundations that provide support for cultural pursuits. Within this chapter, emphasis is directed toward resources that have been given little attention but are essential in assisting the Euro-American elderly. They include the following: the ethnic media, the ethnic elderly or natural helpers, private business, and members of religious bodies.

ETHNIC COMMUNITY RESOURCES

Ethnic Media

Ethnic newspapers, magazines, and radio have functioned historically to provide their audiences with culturally relevant music, news, and articles that foster a sense of belonging and ethnic identity. Today many Euro-American elderly who are limited-English-speaking depend on these media as key information sources for local, national, and international news developments. Each ethnic community has the capacity to reach many Euro-American elderly by utilizing these media as educational tools regarding aging in general, local community resources, and social service procedures and policies. A critical need that could be met by these resources would be to present information on various aspects of aging, older adult service programs, and so forth.

Below is a listing of some ethnic newspapers that have a large elderly readership who could benefit from specific age-related articles.

The Ukrainian Weekly, published since 1933 by the Ukrainian National Association, carries articles ranging in scope from the coverage of local events to commentary on national and international public policy questions. Many of its articles are political in nature, and they focus almost exclusively on events that relate to the Ukrainian community.

The Polish American Voice is published monthly in Buffalo, New York. Its articles focus on various areas, including politics, the humanities, leisure and entertainment, and local events. Although its readership extends well beyond the greater Buffalo area, its advertising indicates that the local Polish community is of primary importance to its publishers. Another topic of great importance is the polka. The paper contains a section of several pages that deals exclusively with polkas, polka bands, polka events, and folklore.

The Northwest Ethnic News, affiliated with the Ethnic Heritage Council of the Pacific Northwest, is multiethnic in character. Distributed from Seattle, Washington, this paper's articles focus mainly on the cultures and traditions of a wide range of ethnic groups in the area. In addition to a variety of articles about the humanities, a monthly calendar of events is published.

Il Progresso Italo-Americano, published in New York City, has both a national and a local edition. Articles focus on national and local events and issues of concern to Italian Americans. *Il Progresso's* circulation in 1977 was 68,637, which represented the largest Italian-language newspaper in print within the United States.

Natural Helpers

Among the most valuable resources in ethnic communities are people called natural helpers, who on a voluntary basis provide assistance to others (Biegel & Sherman, 1979; Quam, 1984). These individuals, who could be family members, neighbors, or friends, have often lived in the ethnic community for years. They often have a strong sense of community pride and in turn are highly regarded and trusted by community residents. Many of them are elderly.

These individuals, who comprise an appreciable segment of our elderly population, can be of great help to their peers because of special talents and abilities. For example, they can provide comfort and support in the native language, help in meal preparation, and deliver assistance in a culturally appropriate manner. Because of their knowledge of the culture and traditions, they often can provide assistance that would not be accepted from a professional. The positive contribution that older Euro-American elderly can make in helping their peers was illustrated by the emotional address of an elderly Hungarian volunteer at the 1985 National Conference on Euro-American Elderly:

> Several years ago an elderly gentleman whom I knew for years called me to be the executor of his will. So I helped him write it, explained it to him, and put it in probate court. Last year he started dying of lung cancer. He had no wife, no family to come and help him. So for a full year I went every day to his house and cooked his meals, gave him medication, and cleaned. When he died, I distributed his $100,000 to different churches and non-profit organizations. He was so grateful to have found someone to take care of him during his last year. . . . Who finds these old people? How do we help them? Can the government do this? No. The churches can't do this [either] because the priest is too busy. Only the community can do this. Old people like myself can talk in the mother tongue. We have the contact to them. They will tell *us* their problems. (Unpublished transcript from National Conference on Euro-American Elderly, 1985)

As natural helpers in ethnic communities the Euro-American elderly act as a critical link between the formal agency structure and the client by (a) identifying ethnic elderly in need of assistance, (b) providing information and referral activity, (c) responding to crisis or emergency situations, and (d) acting as translators and buffers between the agency and the client. In similar roles, previous research studies have found that minority aged, especially neighbors and friends, operated as catalysts and links to the utilization of services and resources (Bell, Kasschau, & Zellman, 1976; Federal Council on the Aging, 1976; Staples, 1976).

It is essential that ethnic communities develop a mechanism to strengthen the capacity of Euro-American elderly to assist their peers on a more formal basis. Writers on aging have recently begun to describe programs that mobilize the voluntary sector by developing or strengthening natural support systems to promote mutual help among older persons. For example, Ehrlich (1979) describes a Mutual Help Model, which organized neighborhood-based groups to encourage socialization and peer group support among older persons who did not use the services of senior centers. Haber (1983) highlights how an educational focus (that is, conferences and short-term training programs) was used to stimulate the organization of mutual help groups. Finally, Ruffini and Todd (1979) utilize a Network Model in which older volunteers identified elderly people on their blocks, distributed newsletters, and provided information and referrals.

The ability of ethnic communities to develop effective programs for their aged may well be determined by the inclusion of the Euro-American elderly as a pivotal resource. Colen and Soto (1979) report from their study of successful programs serving minority aged persons that many of the factors that distinguished successful from unsuccessful programs were highly correlated with the integration of natural helping systems.

Private Business

Private business includes for-profit establishments that range from small grocery stores to giant corporations. Recently, attention has been directed toward the minimal role that private business has played in addressing the needs of the elderly.

> Although it provides by far the most goods and services Americans receive, our private, for-profit sector receives surprisingly little attention in considering ways to meet people's needs, including those of the elderly. We tend to focus on government, though the free enterprise system in most instances is more capable of performing this function. The business sector of our system has the advantage of being able to respond automatically to our changing demands and preferences. It operates without all the difficulties inherent in public programs, such as appropriating the "correct" level of funds, proper targeting, excessive administrative expense, and conformance to a particular political ideology (White House Conference on Aging, 1981).

Today ethnic communities still contain small business establishments such as groceries, produce markets, and restaurants that are operated by immigrant owners who started them many years ago. The resources of these establishments can be utilized in a variety of creative ways to assist, both directly and indirectly, the Euro-American elderly. As an example, many Northeastern urban areas such as Baltimore and New York hold festivals that celebrate the ethnic heritage and culture of a number of Euro-American groups. These events symbolize to the ethnic aged the continuation of cultural traditions and customs that also foster community pride. In addition, they provide opportunities for many Euro-American elderly to demonstrate skills, such as weaving, baking, pottery, arts and crafts, and so forth. Ethnic businesses often donate goods and services to these festivals that provide them with a vehicle to advertise their specific establishments.

The Baltimore Neighborhood Heritage Project clearly illustrates the positive role that private business can play in providing resources to assist ethnic communities and the aged. Organized in 1977 to explore and present in popular form the history of Baltimore as seen through its ethnic neighborhoods, the Baltimore Neighborhood Heritage Project represents a cooperative effort among historians, community leaders, city agencies, and hundreds of ethnic aged. Funded partially through private business, the project supports several activities aimed at involving the public in the pursuit and enjoyment of local history. Activities of the project include (a) community events in which the ethnic aged discuss their life in the neighborhood; (b) a theater group, which presents plays from material obtained through interviews with the ethnic aged; and (c) publications, which discuss different ethnic neighborhoods.

An important question that needs to be examined is whether business can play a role in developing and organizing programs for the Euro-American elderly. To answer this question it is important to point out that some corporate leaders today are either immigrants themselves or were born of immigrant parents. Lopata (1976) describes the "professional and business elites" in the Polish community as the president of Mrs. Paul's Kitchen; the heads of sausage-making firms; and individuals holding high positions in insurance, banking, and the travel industry. These individuals could be approached to assist in developing community-based programs for the Euro-American elderly. An undeniable fact is that these leaders are aging and will become more sensitive to the later stages of life.

Besides providing money, these ethnic corporate leaders should be persuaded to provide resources which assist in developing the foundation for community-based Euro-American elderly programs. Such resources could include the following:

- Loan executives—these individuals could provide expertise in fund raising, management, nonprofit board development, and so forth.
- Board members—corporate leaders and their employees could sit on the board of directors of a nonprofit organization.
- Surplus equipment and supplies—a Euro-American elderly

senior center could be the recipient of donations such as typewriters, food, clothing, and so forth.
- Promotional materials—a newly established ethnic program would need brochures, pamphlets, and information, which could be produced by the company in a number of different languages.

Small business establishments in ethnic communities can also make a significant contribution to the well-being of the Euro-American elderly through (a) providing discounts on merchandise, goods, and services; (b) establishing employment opportunities for those who want to continue working; and (c) making monetary contributions to organizations that attempt to provide outreach and social services.

Members of Religious Bodies

Chapter 7 highlights the important and varying roles that the clergy play in the lives of the Euro-American elderly. However, it is the members of the church (or synagogue) who offer a vast, untapped resource for the Euro-American elderly and their families who need assistance. Many ethnic community churches have as members business and civic leaders, housewives, city employees, and the like, who have remained within the community. These individuals have participated routinely in worship services with older members who may no longer be attending church because of physical disabilities, transportation difficulties, or other problems. It is the author's perspective that church members often lack knowledge regarding the problems associated with old age and are unaware that the elderly are absent from worship services due to special needs.

Church members could play an important role in providing needed services for the Euro-American elderly by organizing recreation/socialization activities, maintaining an informal helping network in the community, initiating and/or developing housing projects, encouraging respite for family caregivers, and organizing translation assistance. The following examples indicate ways that churches have begun to address the needs of elderly Euro-Americans.

- Harvest House is a multi-parish approach to the recreation/ socialization needs of persons over 55 years old in South

Bend, Indiana. St. Adalbert's Parish, one of 28 Harvest House participants, serves a predominantly Polish, moderate-income neighborhood. In addition to masses and various gatherings, this activity group makes special visits to shut-ins, hospitalized members of the community, and those who live in nursing homes. Language barriers do exist for some of the elderly in this community, but there are enough bilingual community members to alleviate this potential problem.

- Our Lady of Czestochowa Parish of Brooklyn, New York, established POMOC, Inc., in the autumn of 1980 in order to deal with a variety of problems in the neighborhood that surrounds the parish. Since that time the parish has provided a number of services to the Polish, Italian, and other eastern European elderly who reside there. These include transportation to medical and social services; assistance with housekeeping, shopping, and meals; and interpreters, when necessary, for some of the older Polish and Italian residents.

To gather the potential that exists within church membership to benefit the Euro-American elderly, the clergy must educate the congregation to the need and develop a mechanism to recruit and organize a program. Religious relief organizations such as Catholic Charities or Jewish Social Services could provide technical assistance to clergy interested in developing programs for the aged. Also, women's and men's organizations that are attached to religious bodies could sponsor a specific program for the Euro-American elderly.

A church-based model that is working in the Hispanic community and has potential for being replicated in Euro-American communities is Project Respeto. Founded 20 years ago, Project Respeto is now in operation in five Los Angeles churches and is slated to be replicated in eight states with large Hispanic populations. The project targets low-income Hispanic elderly who do not take advantage of existing services because of mistrust, a lack of knowledge regarding resources, and language barriers. The basic elements of the program include the following:

- training church-based volunteers of all ages to furnish social supports and services to impaired older persons;
- development of roundtable discussions between Hispanic elderly and youth interested in sharing knowledge, culture, and the arts;

- production of bilingual training and educational materials for use by families and others in furnishing voluntary services to impaired elderly and involving older persons more fully in their communities;
- providing volunteers to families who need a short respite from their caregiving responsibilities.

SERVICES BENEFITING THE EURO-AMERICAN ELDERLY

A variety of ethnic communities throughout the United States have begun to pool available public and private resources to develop programs for the Euro-American elderly. This section is intended to describe a number of those efforts in the hope that they can be replicated and expanded in other ethnic communities. Programs described cover a wide area: information and referral, advocacy, nutrition, housing, and the education of older ethnic women.

There are, however, significant common elements in these programs that must be noted. First, regardless of the program context, each utilizes the Euro-American elderly as an important resource. Each program supports the contention that the ethnic aged are essential ingredients in delivering services. In providing assistance to their peers, the Euro-American elderly gain satisfaction from being contributing members of their community. Second, they have developed strategies that are culturally acceptable, non-threatening, and supported by the ethnic community. Last, all of the projects described have utilized a creative mixture of public and private resources to fund the efforts. It should be noted that because of the brevity of this chapter, not all of the projects that enhance the well-being of the Euro-American elderly could be described.

Outreach and Referral

As mentioned throughout this book, the Euro-American elderly often have difficulty accessing services and benefits because of language barriers, inability to identify community resources, and complicated agency intake procedures. In the projects described in this section, unique outreach techniques have been developed that attempt to help identify isolated Euro-American elderly and provide essential social service information to address their problems. Two programs are described that provide a critical linkage between the formal aging network and the Euro-American aged.

Senior Ethnic Find, Cleveland

Established in 1973 as an ACTION/VISTA project, this program recruits bilingual volunteers to provide linkages between limited-English-speaking or non-English-speaking elderly and service providers. Major activities include

- identification of ethnic elderly who live at or below the poverty level and need some type of community service;
- provision of referrals to appropriate public and private agencies and follow-up studies to ensure service utilization;
- translation of service and benefit information into the necessary Euro-American languages;
- training of professionals and community agencies on the special needs of the Euro-American elderly;
- provision of counseling and home visits to Euro-American elderly in crisis.

The project staff of 22 to 25 individuals is composed of bilingual, older workers who are well known within their own nationality group and community. The following Euro-American communities are served by the project: Croatian, Czech, German, Hungarian, Italian, Polish, Romanian, Serbian, Slovenian, Lithuanian, and Ukrainian. Volunteers are trained to conduct a basic interview, listen effectively, identify local community resources, and make appropriate referrals. Each year the project reaches approximately 5,000 Euro-American elderly who require assistance. Individuals 62 years or older are eligible for program services, and they must live in the city of Cleveland. All services are provided free of charge.

A key to the success of the project is the relative ease with which volunteers gain access to ethnic communities. However, a major problem that the program has faced is funding, which was terminated by ACTION in 1978. The program has continued through minimal city outlays of funds and the dedication of its volunteers, who receive a small stipend and travel reimbursement. In replicating this program elsewhere, Euro-American communities should explore taking some responsibility for the financial basis of the project.

The International Institute, Detroit

This program was initiated in 1984 with a grant from the Detroit Area Agency on Aging to provide bilingual outreach services to the ethnic elderly of eastern European background who live in the Detroit area. The grant provides funding for a social worker who gives translation assistance, counseling, and referral information to Euro-American elderly in four ethnic communities. This staff person has also received training in immigration and naturalization policies and consults routinely with other agency caseworkers regarding the problems of Euro-American elderly.

To be eligible for assistance the client must be at least 60 years of age and of limited English-speaking ability. Low-income, handicapped, or isolated Euro-American elderly are given priority. The program is able to provide assistance to more than 100 Euro-American elderly per year.

A related program that is being established by the International Institute is called the Ethnic Connection. It is a telephone reassurance program specializing in eastern European languages. Ethnic aged volunteers will be recruited to contact by telephone isolated or vulnerable Euro-American elderly. These volunteers will receive training in basic social work techniques, the aging process, and available community resources. Each Euro-American elderly person who requests the service will be called daily by an older volunteer who is fluent in the common language.

Advocacy

It is the contention of this author that only through advocacy and political action can ethnic communities develop needed social services for the aged. Certain ethnic organizations have combined the task of providing needed services to their aged and at the same time advocate for the necessary funding to expand their efforts. One such organization that satisfies both requirements is described below.

United Polish American Services, Philadelphia

The United Polish American Social Services (PASS) provides assistance to the city's Polish community. PASS is dedicated to the idea that cultural obstacles to receiving services can be overcome through professional and sensitive outreach and political advocacy. The following services are provided:

- social service information and referral in Polish and English;
- assistance in completing rebate, senior citizen discount, and various other eligibility forms;
- translation services for those with language barriers;
- assistance in dealing with public and private agencies, programs, departments, and so forth;
- home visitations to the handicapped elderly;
- information and news in English and Polish via flyers, newsletters, Polish-American radio programs, local newspapers, and speaking engagements.

In 1985 PASS provided assistance to 2,100 elderly Polish Americans in the city of Philadelphia. The staff is composed of seven full-time and seven part-time employees, as well as volunteers. Funding for PASS is received from city and state sources. To date its most notable achievement is advocating for the Euro-American Ethnic and Multicultural Social Services Act, a bill introduced in the General Assembly of Pennsylvania, to provide funding for

> . . . grants by the Secretary of Community Affairs to promote government-related social services for Pennsylvania's ethnic and multicultural heritage and to insure that ethnic groups are not discriminated against or prohibited from receiving services because of language barriers, cultural obstacles, lack of education or lack of accessibility to government-related or public social programs. (General Assembly of Pennsylvania, 1985).

The bill would appropriate $2 million for grants to social service agencies interested in addressing the social service needs of the ethnic individual within the state of Pennsylvania. According to a PASS spokesperson, other ethnic organizations could advocate for similar bills within their particular state.

Nutrition

The nutrition program for older adults, authorized under the Older Americans Act, has been acclaimed as one of the most popular and well-received programs of the 1970s (Gelfand, 1984). Under this program older adults receive a nutritious meal in a congregate setting, socialize, and obtain needed social services. However, the Congregate Nutrition Program has been criticized for not developing specific outreach efforts to increase ethnic/minority representation within the service (U.S. Civil Rights Commission, 1982). Within the last several years attempts have been made to place nutrition sites strategically within ethnic/minority communities and provide more culturally appropriate services. The nutrition project described below is specifically addressing the unique needs of the ethnic aged and developing strategies to attract large numbers of Euro-American older adults into the program.

Eating Together in Baltimore

Eating Together in Baltimore, sponsored by the Baltimore City Health Department, is an effort to improve the health and well-being of older adults in the following ways:

- providing nutritious meals in a group setting;
- fostering social interaction;
- presenting nutrition education programs concerning the kinds and amounts of food required to satisfy nutritional requirements;
- assisting in obtaining food stamps, Social Security benefits, homemaker services, legal advice, Medicare, and shopping aid.

The program, funded through the Older Americans Act, has placed its 70 nutrition sites strategically in areas with large concentrations of ethnic aged. Efforts were made to place sites so that no older adult has more than a few blocks to walk. Because of the wide diversity in the older population of Baltimore and the large numbers of Euro-American elderly, special attention is placed on ethnicity. For example, older adults have direct input into menu planning, which reflects the cuisine of various cultures. Entertainment and social events at the sites often are oriented around cultural traditions and customs. In addition, participants are encouraged to become volunteers in conducting outreach to the ethnic community and providing needed information regarding social services.

Each year the program serves approximately 130,000 meals to Euro-American elderly. Eating Together in Baltimore illustrates the potential for developing culturally appropriate services by engaging the ethnic aged to become an integral part of the program.

Housing

Affordable housing for the elderly has become a national issue. Today, roughly 2 million low-income elderly renters who are eligible for federal housing assistance are not served by federal programs. This problem is expected to continue as the numbers of older Americans increase, and the cost of housing rises in relation to other living expenses (U.S. Senate Special Committee on Aging, 1984). Especially problematic for many ethnic aged is that available public housing is not oriented toward providing an atmosphere in which language, culture, and traditions are compatible. At this time many ethnic communities are questioning how they can provide housing for their aged who want to continue their cultural identity during their later years. The housing project described below is one ethnic community's response to the need.

Ukrainian Village, Warren, MI

In 1965 the Detroit District Regional Council of the Ukrainian National Women's League of America (Soyuz Ukrainok) formed a building fund committee to develop a housing project for elderly Ukrainians in the Detroit area. Guided by a cadre of housing activists, the group received more than $100,000 in donations and land for the project. Recognizing that private funds would not be enough to construct a housing complex, the group submitted an application to the U.S. Housing and Urban Development Agency (HUD) under Section 202 for a low-interest loan. After being rejected once, the group filed a second application and on September 23, 1982, received a $6,737,000 loan to build housing for the elderly. Ukrainian Village has gained national recognition and has become the model for other ethnic groups interested in building housing for their aged. The Village includes

- a two-story residence with 146 individual units located on 7 acres of land;
- a geographical location that is uniquely cradled among hundreds of Ukrainian homes, St. Josaphat's Ukrainian Catholic Church, a two-story Ukrainian Cultural Center, and a Ukrainian Village Plaza (unrelated to the Ukrainian Village) that encloses a Camopomich Center replete with Ukrainian artifacts and a federal credit union called the Ukrainian Selfreliance;

- 15 units for handicapped elderly;
- resident volunteers who provide lunches once a week.

According to Anastasia Volker, president of Ukrainian Village, there is a growing realization that the elderly need to congregate with people of their own cultural backgrounds and form their social and community life within these complexes. In Detroit many Euro-American communities are now building housing for their elderly so that they may continue life surrounded by cultural familiarity. The need for ethnic housing is tremendous, and more communities will need to take a leadership role in the future.

Ethnic Women

Ethnic women's attitudes toward aging often depend on the role models they have—mothers, aunts, other older women in the community. These role models have traditionally communicated that a woman's vocation is one of caretaker even if one has a job outside of the family. This sense of responsibility is placing heavy burdens on middle-aged and older ethnic women who are often the caretakers for frail spouses and sick family members. Since many ethnic women have had to return to work due to economic necessity, they find it difficult to juggle caregiving and paid employment.

Many ethnic women are looking for guidance and direction to help them cope with the realities of caregiving. In addition, there is a critical need to prepare midlife ethnic women to face potential health, economic, and employment issues in old age. The project described below attempts to educate ethnic women regarding old age and to develop strategies to address future potential problems.

Facing Our Future: A Unique Educational Program for Mid-Life Working-Class Women, Washington, DC

Started initially from a Department of Education grant, Facing Our Future is geared toward working-class or lower-middle-class women in ethnic communities. The concept of the project is to provide information regarding age-related issues and at the same time foster support networks. Because many ethnic women feel threatened by professional caregivers, the project uses a peer counseling concept in presenting information. To provide these women with a comfortable environment where they can articulate their needs and be accepted, churches, community buildings, and labor union sites are used.

An important part of the package that was developed for Facing Our Future are audiotape presentations of women speaking honestly and openly about aging, emotional issues that arise in midlife, health, and finances. The voices heard are ethnic and minority women from all over the United States, including neighborhood women from Brooklyn, Chicago, and San Francisco. The tapes create a climate that validates the participants' personal experiences and values and stimulates discussions about personal options and choices. The program is designed to be peer-led, and a 200-page *Leader's Manual* gives detailed directions for implementing the learning activities. Information is conveyed through these activities and through sharing ideas and resources.

Each participant receives a manual with worksheets, quizzes, games, and activities for the sessions. Simple charts and clear narratives are included to reinforce information presented during the sessions and to serve as a resource for the future. Resources easily obtainable from other organizations also are listed.

The program is designed to be used in small groups of 10 to 20 women. The six sessions are 2 hours long and can be held once a week or in a weekend workshop format. The sessions cover attitudes on aging, health, finances, education, employment, and emotional health. Facing Our Future promotes positive attitudinal changes about women and the aging process; provides information on health, finances (Social Security, pensions, IRAs, Medicare, and so forth), education, employment, and emotional concerns; develops planning skills; and brings about behavioral changes through mutual support.

The program was tested in a wide variety of sites throughout the country, including churches, ethnic women's organizations, labor unions, and community groups. The response was extremely favorable in every case. Jo Vanden Berg, who led Facing Our Future at St. Robert Bellarmine's Parish in Flushing, Michigan, stated, "We are so grateful that this program was designed; it is truly filling a need. Our women learned so much" (personal communication).

CONCLUSION

This chapter has presented some ideas regarding untapped ethnic community resources and a number of model projects aimed at enhancing the well-being of the Euro-American elderly. In analyzing the projects described above, a variety of critical issues arises. First, these programs have succeeded due to innovative funding strategies that gather resources from within the ethnic community itself and utilize public support if available. These programs demonstrate that ethnic communities can capitalize on both their own resources and those of the larger society. Simultaneously, ethnic communities must take inventory of what can be provided in-house to develop aging services along with securing governmental funding.

Second, these programs should demonstrate to government funding bodies that providing resources toward self-help efforts can strengthen an ethnic community's capacity to provide assistance to the aged. None of the programs highlighted could survive without some form of government assistance, but at the same time, their impact would be greatly diminished without resources in the ethnic community such as volunteers and donated services. It is imperative that cooperative efforts continue to be established between ethnic communities and government funding bodies such as the Area Agencies on Aging (AAAs). As noted in the International Institute project, the AAA is an instrumental funding figure in developing culturally appropriate services for the Euro-American elderly. Such advisory bodies as the National Association of Area Agencies on Aging should explore how more AAAs can play important roles in fostering self-help movements in ethnic communities on behalf of the Euro-American aged.

Third, a number of these programs symbolize the importance of advocacy in ensuring that the Euro-American elderly receive public benefits. In many of these programs it was one individual who acted as a catalyst in lobbying state and city government officials for the needed legislation or funding. In recent years several ethnic organizations have claimed that the Euro-American aged have not received their fair share of public benefits and services. These resources will be obtained only through concerted advocacy efforts. As these programs demonstrate, the system will provide resources, but they must be obtained through raising the concerns of the Euro-American elderly in a patient, consistent, unbending manner.

Last, the Euro-American elderly themselves stand as the most important resource in providing support to their peers. More attention needs to be given to the ways in which ethnic communities can build on this resource in formulating programs and services.

11

The Need for Collaboration among Religious, Ethnic, and Public Service Institutions

Christopher L. Hayes, Ph.D., and David Guttmann, D.S.W.

Today a growing recognition is emerging in society of the cross-cutting, multifaceted needs of older people. This awareness, coupled with economic and political considerations, is requiring public and private entities to work together toward the common goals of enhancing the well-being of the elderly. As Froland, Pancoast, Chapman, and Kimboko (1981) noted, it seems clear that no one source of care, be it public, private, or voluntary, can by itself adequately meet the needs of dependent populations.

Religious and ethnic community institutions play a central role in the lives of the ethnic aged (Fandetti & Gelfand, 1976; Naparstek, Biegel, & Spence, 1978; Guttmann et al., 1979a). A collaborative approach between these entities, in concert with available public resources, holds potential for providing comprehensive services for the Euro-American elderly. This contention is based on research on the Euro-American elderly which shows that these community institutions are central in the lives of the ethnic aged.

To assist the Euro-American elderly, religious and ethnic organizational leadership must first become familiar with the basic needs of survival that affect their elderly (income maintenance, health care, adequate housing, and so forth). Once this is done, ethnic leaders can play a vital role by both informing their elderly of the existence of services within the community to meet these needs and assisting them in gaining access to these resources. Similar to the church (synagogues and Protestant and Catholic churches are included throughout when we use *church*), an ethnic organization has the potential for mediating between the sometimes impersonal bureaucracies of social service agencies and the ethnic older adult. The ethnic organization could act as an advocate to ensure that needs are met in accordance with the traditions and customs of the community.

Many ethnic communities are too small and lack the resources to develop *ethnic elderly–specific* projects. For these communities, collaborative efforts with other institutions, such as the church, can be indispensable for assisting the needy elderly among them.

This chapter will offer a rationale for developing a model for collaboration among religious, ethnic, and public service institutions. A basic assumption is that collaborative efforts between church or synagogue, ethnic, and government-sponsored programs to address the needs of Euro-American elderly are a necessity. *Collaboration,* as used in this chapter, is defined as working jointly with others, or cooperating with an agency or institution with which one is not immediately connected (Webster's Seventh New Collegiate Dictionary, 1971). Such efforts could include the sharing of resources, developing common objectives, and/or coordinating services for an identified group. However, as Estes (1979) points out, collaboration between public and private institutions rarely occurs.

We will limit our discussion to four questions that need to be answered before presenting our model for collaboration among the entities cited above:

1. Why should the mediating structures in the ethnic community collaborate?
2. What are the barriers at the community level that may prevent collaboration from occurring?
3. What research evidence is available to support our contention?
4. What are the main elements of a working model for collaboration of the mediating structures in the ethnic community?

WHY SHOULD THE MEDIATING STRUCTURES IN THE ETHNIC COMMUNITY COLLABORATE?

Several reasons can be given why the coordination of mediating structures is essential. First, the present Euro-American elderly population is composed of individuals born around the turn of the century. This population will invariably need more assistance such as chore services, meal preparation, and so forth, as they approach the old-old (the term used by gerontologists to designate people 85 years of age or older who generally need a number of health care services) category. Family members may not be able to provide all of the in-home supportive assistance needed by the elderly due to financial and geographic constraints. Some Euro-American elderly may not have any family to provide such aid. Because of language barriers and cultural obstacles the Euro-American elderly will need mediating structures that can provide follow-up and intervention when assistance is not forthcoming from the formal social service system. Therefore, to keep this group from being prematurely institutionalized, community resources will have to be generated as existing services are severely strained. According to the National Conference on Social Welfare (1977), 60% of the people who seek social services are turned away from agencies. The church and ethnic organizations will be increasingly called on to provide services to those elderly whose needs go unaddressed by existing social service agencies. Collaborative efforts among religious, ethnic, and public service institutions can blend resources that will be needed to address the burgeoning old-old population.

Second, due to the reduction of funds from public resources and the increase in service demand, there will be a need to utilize informal support systems more effectively than in the past. It has been estimated that only one of five people referred from one service to another ever reaches the agency to which they are referred (National Conference on Social Welfare, 1977). If the church and ethnic organizations established greater collaboration among them for assisting the elderly, then more individuals would benefit from services offered by existing public agencies.

Third, public and philanthropic funding sources are requiring that communities develop coordinative efforts in addressing human needs. Quite common today are foundations that solicit proposals from urban communities in order to coordinate model service programs for the elderly among public, private, and voluntary institutions. It is obvious that a united front—an agreement among religious, ethnic, and public entities—will be mutually beneficial in securing funding for the needs of the Euro-American elderly.

The following case illustration provides an example of how public, ethnic, and religious institutions can work together: A 78-year-old Hungarian immigrant is in crisis due to her inability to understand why she is being evicted from her apartment. She has no family, and she turns to her pastor for guidance. In today's situation it is possible that the pastor does not understand Hungarian. However, he may contact a representative from the local Hungarian-American Community Center for assistance. After a translator is provided, the woman is able to explain clearly in her native tongue the problems she has been having with her landlord. In responding to the woman's crisis, the Hungarian-American Community Center provides emotional support through daily visits to the home as the pastor works with the local Area Agency on Aging to identify potential city housing projects for senior citizens.

If we analyze the above situation, the elderly Hungarian immigrant was able to receive assistance because of the unique qualities of each of the three institutions involved. The church represents a natural assistance institution for ethnic elderly in crisis, which is not associated with public welfare and does not involve elaborate intake procedures as a prerequisite for obtaining aid. Similarly, the ethnic organization contains members who not only can assist with translation but have intimate knowledge of cultural life-styles and customs that can be particularly helpful in assisting with a crisis. Last, the Area Agency on Aging has information and resources that can be critical in resolving social service concerns of the elderly.

How Often Do We Witness Such Collaboration between Institutions within Our Ethnic Communities?

There is relatively little information or research concerning the extent to which religious, ethnic, and public service institutions are conducting collaborative efforts on behalf of the Euro-American elderly. To gain further knowledge regarding such efforts, the staff of The Catholic University of America's Center for the Study of Pre-Retirement and Aging conducted a survey that was administered to ethnic leaders, clergy, and service providers at the National Conference on Euro-American Elderly in 1985. Of 125 participants who were given the questionnaire, only 42 who returned the questionnaire completed it. Although the findings are limited to those who filled out the questionnaire, we cite them because they may be valuable in future efforts to study more carefully the collaboration among religious, ethnic, and public service institutions. The survey results indicated that:

1. Ethnic organizations varied dramatically concerning the extent to which they were aware of problems faced by their elderly or the need to coordinate such assistance with religious or public institutions.
2. Few respondents could identify any allied approaches among ethnic, religious, or public service institutions.
3. Efforts to assist the Euro-American elderly by the above-mentioned institutions were often conducted without formal assistance from the Area Agency on Aging.

Some ethnic communities are more sensitive than others to the need for collaboration in addressing the problems of the ethnic elderly. In certain areas of the country special programs have been developed to coordinate assistance, such as Senior Ethnic Find in Cleveland, Ohio (see Chapter 10). Unfortunately, many ethnic communities have not taken an inventory of their available resources for assisting older Euro-Americans in crisis. Ethnic communities do not need to build new programs specifically for their elderly, but rather to utilize what is currently available in building a support system for the aged. Dr. David Biegel has stated:

> Our social service system has failed to understand the concept of community and has ignored neighborhoods and their support systems. I believe the answer to these issues is not, as many would have us believe, a program approach involving another new program or another new service. Rather, these issues can best be addressed through a process that utilizes the naturally occurring strengths and resources in ethnic communities. The elements of community support systems are varied. They include: the woman in her 60's on the block that neighbors turn to for help or support when their welfare checks are late; the clergyman that parishioners talk to about family problems; and the ethnic organization that helps the middle-aged parents with the strains caused by value conflicts with their children. . . . Thus, family, friends, neighbors, co-workers, clergy, neighborhood organizations, and mutual aid groups can all provide meaningful assistance in times of need. (Testimony of Dr. David Beigel before the U.S. Civil Rights Commission, 1979, pp. 312–317)

Combining the church, ethnic organization, and Area Agency on Aging into one organized community support system has great potential for assisting the Euro-American elderly. Such an alignment of collaborating resources could offer help to the ethnic aged in a culturally acceptable manner without stigma or loss of pride. The Euro-American elderly seeking help would not need to identify themselves as having a problem, being weak or sick—a client or a patient—as they would if seeking help from a social service agency or government-sponsored program.

WHAT ARE THE BARRIERS AT THE COMMUNITY LEVEL THAT MAY PREVENT COLLABORATION FROM OCCURRING?

The U.S. Conference of Mayors (1982) indicated that barriers to collaboration at the community level are often based on constraints of law, regulations, or authority, whereas other barriers may be caused by local customs, professional conflicts, personalities, and/or politics. "Many agencies working in isolation fail to adequately communicate with other community agencies which could complement and strengthen their efforts. Some agencies tend to focus too narrowly on their own particular program and take action to 'protect' what they perceive as their 'turf'" (p. 8).

Tobin and Ellor (1983) have identified a variety of reasons why clergy do not usually collaborate with other churches and social service agencies. These are (a) theological differences, (b) lack of lay leadership, (c) lack of resources, (d) demands on an already busy schedule, and (e) lack of awareness concerning other community resources. However, churches and the religious sector in general are slowly beginning to realize that they do not have the financial resources, extensive staff, nor lay support needed to reach all the unmet needs and must utilize other community resources in assisting their congregations.

Ethnic organizations and communities have their own barriers to overcome if collaboration with outside local institutions is to take place. Besides the obvious barrier involving a general lack of knowledge concerning what constitutes the aging network and how to interface with it, ethnic leaders often do not trust the system and do not believe that it really cares about their needs. This lack of faith often leads to complacency and resignation. For example, at the National Conference on Euro-American Elderly held in Washington, DC in 1985 a Ukrainian leader indicated that her organization has tried for five years to no avail to gain financial support from the Area Agency on Aging. "I'm not sure we can continue the fight much longer," she exclaimed. "We simply are running out of patience and energy." Brown (1984) explains how a group such as the one identified above, addresses perceived barriers:

- It is difficult for one group to believe that others will support its agenda. Some differences among groups have been used to justify a group's inhumane treatment and persecution of others.
- Some groups suffer internal fragmentation and friction. A history of persecution may result in members' disagreeing on how to address the problem.
- Some groups find an excuse to maintain isolation. Because isolation is familiar and therefore seems safe, groups sometimes react to a barrier through withdrawal.
- Groups may unintentionally frustrate their best allies. Even after trying very hard to ally themselves with another group, a group or individual occasionally becomes a target of the other's resentment for past years of disappointment and mistreatment.

Models of Collaboration in Operation

It would be a miscalculation on our part to believe that the barriers outlined above can be easily addressed. However, we have found ethnic communities in such cities as Seattle and Chicago that have fostered collaborative efforts between divergent institutions with the goal of both raising ethnic awareness and fostering social service collaboration. For example, the Ethnic Heritage Council in Seattle, Washington, was founded in 1981 to address the problems of isolated Euro-American elderly. Recognizing the need to utilize the resources and talents of different public, private, and ethnic groups to assist the Euro-American elderly, a small group of 11 individuals formulated a model to bring these entities together.

The foundation of this model is a monthly forum that is held within different ethnic communities in the Seattle area. The purpose of these forums is to give public officials, social service providers, clergy, and other interested individuals an opportunity to hear presentations regarding a particular ethnic group's culture, life-style, and concerns. The audience has an opportunity both to discuss the problems presented and to brainstorm about solutions. By bringing different groups together, the Ethnic Heritage Council believes that they are breaking down myths and stereotypes that often impede dialogue between different ethnic and public/private organizations. Since the inception of the program their accomplishments have been impressive.

Since 1984 the Ethnic Heritage Council has published a newspaper called *The Northwest Ethnic,* which describes both the ethnic groups in the community and the goals of the organization. With the assistance of the Seattle Public Library, an ethnic directory was published that lists more than 300 organizations with contact persons and describes the goals of the group as well as the assistance provided. The Seattle–King County Area Agency on Aging assisted in distribution of the document to help service providers identify ethnic resources when addressing Euro-American elders in crisis. To sensitize the Seattle public to the different ethnic groups in the city, the Ethnic Heritage Council has also produced, with the cooperation of local merchants, an "Eat Ethnic" restaurant coupon book.

In evaluating other successful collaborative efforts between diverse community entities that benefit the elderly, the National Council on Aging (1981) found the following concepts to be essential:

- Team leadership—from each cooperating entity there must be decision-making representatives who help set goals and objectives.
- Open-mindedness—each entity must have a willingness and desire to compromise, negotiate, and give up "turf protection." The representatives must look toward the final impact, not just the current problems.
- Ability to recognize status—participants should be able to recognize weaknesses and strengths and work toward developing mutual contributions.
- Willingness to take responsibility—each decision-maker must take responsibility for his/her home agency support team and agree to work out problems in-house.
- Consensus of ground rules—operating rules should be established in early development stages to minimize straying from goals and objectives.

- Agreement on concept—no one member of the team is as smart or as effective as the whole team.

Leadership

Collaboration is often difficult to achieve due to the large numbers and varieties of people involved in different institutions. Collaboration between different institutions is often accidental—a function of two people who know each other or one person who takes the initiative and opens a line of communication between key decision-makers. The issue of who is responsible for taking a leadership role in making collaboration happen is an important one. Leadership is an essential requirement in any effective operation.

Ethnic communities that wish to explore collaborative efforts must answer the following questions: (a) who should establish a leadership role in fostering collaboration? (b) what local agency is responsible for coordinating services for the elderly? (c) what leadership structures in ethnic communities should be tapped in seeking collaboration?

Answers to the above questions will vary from community to community. However, several key suggestions can be offered to address the leadership issue. An important local agency responsible for coordinating services for the elderly is the Area Agency on Aging (AAA). The AAA is statutorily required to develop a comprehensive and coordinated system of services. This entity can play a critical leadership function by either initiating or responding to a request to explore such an effort. The following points illustrate the many leadership roles that AAA can play in fostering collaboration:

- exercise coordinative powers in support of efforts to include religious institutions and ethnic organizations as part of the aging network;
- establish and maintain effective working relationships with the mediating structures within ethnic communities;
- reinforce efforts to expand religious and ethnic institutional involvement in service planning for the Euro-American elderly;
- provide central leadership for efforts to provide funding to older adult services that are culturally appropriate.

Both religious and ethnic organizations have important leadership structures that can be tapped for collaborative efforts. As noted in the chapter on religion, the pastor or rabbi is a central figure to be utilized in developing services and negotiating with outside entities. If this individual is too overburdened with other responsibilities, a member of the church could be utilized.

Ethnic organizations often have women's groups that could be approached about initiating or developing a collaborative effort. The reader will note in Chapter 10 that most programs assisting the Euro-American elderly have been initiated by women. It is the author's observation that ethnic women within these organizations seem to be more sensitive to the concerns of the elderly and more willing to organize specific social service efforts.

Suggested Model for Collaboration among Ethnic, Religious, and Public Sector Institutions

Our model for collaboration is based on a series of interrelated steps that, taken into consideration prior to engaging in various activities, may generate increased resources.

Obviously, a community is composed of many different groups and leadership structures. The model below is intended to assist either a particular ethnic group or a coalition of various ethnic groups in developing an organized effort to assist the Euro-American elderly within a given community. The model presented is flexible and can be adapted to ensure that the needs of a community's Euro-American elderly population are adequately addressed. The only requirement of the model is that an individual implementing it has patience, time, and a desire to advocate on behalf of the Euro-American elderly.

Developing a Small Working Group

Identify individuals from ethnic and religious groups, and senior citizen service providers who are either interested in reaching out to the Euro-American elderly or are currently engaged in such an activity. These individuals could include a clergyman who provides assistance within a largely ethnic congregation, a Polish administrator of a local board and care home, or a leader of the Sons of Italy chapter in your city. It is important to find persons who are particularly knowledgeable about the problems of the ethnic elderly and are aware of the senior service system within the community. In developing this working group, it is very important to attempt to find several Euro-Americans who can speak from experience about the problems facing this group.

Formulating a Needs/Resource Plan

Meet monthly to draft a document that details the particular contributions that Euro-American elders make in your community. Highlight the unique social service concerns that the ethnic elderly in your community face, such as affordable housing, translation assistance, and so on. If the document attempts to address various Euro-American elderly concerns, be sure to circulate the document to knowledgeable members for input.

Developing a Euro-American Elderly Impact Strategy

After identifying both the contributions and needs of your community's Euro-American elderly population, formulate a strategy that identifies and answers the following questions: (a) what does this working group want to accomplish in 1, 2, or 5 years? (b) what groups or organizations have a vested interest in addressing the working group's goals? (c) how can divergent groups be motivated to assist while at the same time respecting the cultural and religious perspectives of others? (d) what resources need to be generated to implement the group's goals?

Organizing a Community Program

After a plan of action is formulated, the community and its accompanying institutions need to be made aware of what has been developed. However, a word of caution is in order here. We can assume that the level of awareness concerning the issues affecting the Euro-American elderly will vary dramatically. In addition, certain groups may be resistant to participating in any proposal that involves another ethnic group. To share the working group's plans and to lower resistance, we recommend holding a community program that is positive in nature and highlights the contributions of different European groups to the community. Ultimately, ethnic groups participate in a multiethnic function only to the extent that they can be encouraged to be proud of their history and achievements. The goals of the working group can be woven into the fabric of the program as a secondary agenda item. It must be kept in mind that the overall goal of developing a community meeting is to bring diverse ethnic groups together so that they can collaborate in ways of relating to one another. This can act as a springboard for addressing the larger goal of focusing ethnic resources on the needs of the community's ethnic immigrant elderly.

Strengthening Institutional Communication, Resource Provision, and Referral

One hopes the community meeting will build trust among ethnic groups and raise the level of awareness concerning the Euro-American elderly. Follow-up meetings should be conducted with ethnic leaders, service providers, and clergy who can offer resources and assistance to Euro-American elderly in crisis. Attention should be given to how the ethnic community can both utilize the identified existing resources and ensure that communication channels are clearly established between referral sources. Any information gathered during this collaborative building phase should be coordinated and channeled through the county's AAA information and referral office. Such information concerning potential ethnic resources which are culturally appropriate for Euro-American elderly can bolster the AAA's capacity to respond to referrals from the locality's social service providers.

Implementing an Ongoing Monitoring System and Continued Support

Once referrals are being made between ethnic institutions and religious/social service entities, it is critical that such efforts continue and are provided with ongoing support. The working group that acted as a catalyst for this collaborative effort will probably not have the resources to act as an ongoing monitoring system to ensure that information, assistance, and referrals are crossing ethnic institutional lines. Thus, a city's Council on Senior Citizens or some formalized neutral body would be an ideal sponsor to continue hosting meetings between ethnic organizations and religious/social service providers. This effort is doomed to failure unless the collaborative process delineates a structure of responsibility for the effort.

CONCLUSION

This chapter has addressed issues related to collaboration among groups such as clergy, ethnic organizations, and service providers as a necessity for successfully addressing the needs of elderly Euro-Americans. Such collaboration is necessitated by the realization that in today's complex world no one agency or institution, no matter how strong or resourceful, can meet the needs of the Euro-American elderly. Furthermore, there are inherent strengths and resources available in each organization that require a willingness on the part of their leaders to accomplish this function. The authors are not ignorant of the fact that collaboration presents a unique effort, and those engaged in such efforts usually encounter barriers that may at times seem almost insurmountable. In particular, there is a need to dissolve the atmosphere of suspicion and mistrust, and to overcome tendencies of isolation. Models for successfully negotiating the difficulties involved in collaboration among the parties have been presented for consideration. Ethnic communities have a unique opportunity to help the elderly by linking culturally appropriate forms of assistance and existing social service resources into a unified approach to problems in the ethnic community. Such an approach entails finding ways to foster trust within and among ethnic communities and groups and to discover collaborative models that support mutual listening and sharing between institutions. We must also recognize that true collaboration requires a commitment to sharing available resources.

At present, it is too early to say how many specific collaborative programs for the Euro-American elderly will result from such efforts. However, we can identify critical strategies that foster communication between different ethnic, public, private, and religious institutions. These are (a) sharing of cultural strengths, (b) educating the public regarding ethnic diversity, (c) fostering both social and economic cooperative efforts that benefit the ethnic community, and (d) dissemination of material that describes the components that make up an ethnic community.

The main elements of the model presented in this paper for achieving this objective include developing small working groups, formulating a needs/resource plan, developing an impact strategy, organizing a community program, strengthening institutional communication, and implementing an ongoing monitoring system and continued support. This model may be workable, especially for Euro-American elderly who have no family support. We believe that this model has the potential to become a successful one, especially when it is used creatively.

12

The Need for Education and Training*

Christopher L. Hayes, Ph.D., Joseph Giordano, M.S.W., and Irving M. Levine, B.S.

The training and education of professionals regarding the concerns of the Euro-American elderly are essential prerequisites for improving the delivery of social services to this group. Service providers have much to gain through educational opportunities that highlight the role of ethnicity in both delivering and accepting assistance. It is our contention that the recognized failure of the aging network to respond to Euro-American elderly concerns is due partly to lack of professional awareness and of appropriate skills and knowledge.

During the last decade great strides have been made to train service providers to deliver services to the minority aged. The Administration on Aging has funded a number of minority aging centers at academic institutions to facilitate such training opportunities. Much of the training has focused on the generally recognized minority groups (Blacks, Hispanics, Asian Americans) with little attention directed toward the Euro-American elderly. Although the 1981 White House Mini-Conference on Euro-American Elderly strongly recommended increased training for service providers and religious personnel regarding the delivery of services to ethnic elderly subgroups, little progress has been made.

*The training principles and models discussed in this chapter were developed at the Center on Ethnicity, Behavior, and Communications, and the Institute for American Pluralism of the American Jewish Committee.

A basic assumption of this chapter is that minority aging training programs need to expand their focus to include the concerns of the Euro-American elderly. A multiethnic perspective in training gerontologists will provide agencies with the ability to address a wide array of groups that surround the community. As community-based services continue to be strained because of a diminished amount of funds, professionals will be forced to expand their efforts in working with a variety of ethnic groups. Our perspective is that gerontologists need to be trained adequately to address the different needs of ethnic groups.

In an attempt to remedy this deficiency, this chapter presents fundamental concepts and recommends specific models that can be utilized in training professionals and students in working with the Euro-American elderly. The following questions will be addressed:

1. What should be the role of the service agency, Area Agency on Aging, and academic institutions in training present and future gerontologists regarding Euro-American elderly issues?
2. What basic principles and ethnocultural factors need to be incorporated into training models?
3. What problems can trainers expect in providing training on ethnicity?
4. What resources can a trainer draw on in developing in-service sessions concerning ethnicity and aging?
5. What strategies can be implemented on a national level that would ensure ongoing training efforts regarding Euro-American elderly concerns?

THE ROLE OF SERVICE ORGANIZATIONS AND ACADEMIC INSTITUTIONS

Although some social service agencies may be providing specific training opportunities for staff on the unique concerns of the Euro-American aged, we have found this to be the exception rather than the rule. We can identify a number of factors that historically have impeded training and education efforts to bolster an organization's capacity to work with the Euro-American elderly. First, few training models exist to sensitize gerontology professionals regarding ethnocultural factors in service delivery to this group. A director of a senior center who wishes to educate staff on conducting outreach to the Euro-American community would be hard-pressed to identify an existing training model.

Second, despite the importance of ethnicity in the delivery of services to the elderly, ethnicity is not emphasized sufficiently within agency in-service training sessions (Giordano & Levine, 1984). Often, few formal opportunities occur to facilitate such awareness due to fear, stereotypical thinking, and a lack of an agencywide commitment to such an effort. Failing to develop formalized efforts to raise ethnic and cultural sensitivity among staff can have a detrimental effect on the quality of care provided. As an example, the *New York Times* on June 17, 1983, ran a story on the conflicts that arose between patients and staff in New York City nursing homes due to ethnic differences.

Third, most professionals providing services under the Older Americans Act rely on the Area Agency on Aging for training and workshops to increase age-related knowledge. According to the National Association of Area Agencies on Aging (NAAAA), Area Agencies vary in the extent to which they have formalized strategies in training service providers regarding ethnic issues. For many Area Agencies, ethnic training for service providers is not occurring due to limited training resources within the Older Americans Act:

> Title IV training dollars have been gradually reduced over the past decade. As priorities at the federal level change, so will the priorities at subsequent levels. Since the Older Americans Act does not mandate ethnic training at the local level, Area Agencies are not forced to support or encourage it with local providers. Ethnic training is simply not a priority of the Act or the Administration today. (Glendale V. Wiggins, personal communication, October 29, 1985)

Several Area Agencies on Aging have taken a leadership role in training gerontology professionals regarding minority issues. Similar efforts should be developed to expand the training to include the Euro-American elderly. For example, the Pike's Peak Area Agency on Aging in Colorado Springs, Colorado, contracted with the Medical Care and Research Foundation in Denver to develop a "Minority Outreach Training Manual" to assist the agency in training local service providers to better serve the Black and Hispanic elderly of the Colorado Springs area. As a resource manual, it provides background information on the cultural and ethnic characteristics of Black and Hispanic subpopulations. As a training manual, it contains information related to actual training—process, content, and method.

In a similar effort the New York City Department of Aging instituted the Minority Service Enhancement Project, which involved holding a series of workshops for the Department's professional and volunteer staff. Each workshop attempted to raise the level of awareness of the ways in which ethnocultural factors impact on service delivery.

During the last decade a fair number of academic institutions have developed specialized curricula and courses that focus on ethnicity and aging. For example, the National Catholic School of Social Service (NCSSS) at The Catholic University of America has been in the vanguard of including in professional education an appreciation of ethnic pluralism. In 1977, NCSSS received a grant from the U.S. Department of Health, Education, and Welfare to develop "teaching modules" on ethnicity for inclusion in a variety of curricular areas. Since this early work, several innovative approaches have been made to extend ethnicity and aging education beyond its inclusion in general social work courses.

The University of Kansas has developed a gerontological course on ethnicity and aging that also engages students to work directly with ethnic elderly. The students read extensively about a particular cultural group, then invite a panel of ethnic elderly to discuss how they perceive old age, their health practices, and what they expect from service providers. Taking on the role of teacher gives self-esteem and recognition to the elderly, and at the same time sensitizes students to ethnocultural factors in service provision.

The introduction of the effect of ethnocultural factors on services for the aged into training programs may be initiated on different levels. It may reflect an agency-wide or institutional commitment; it may be funded by an outside source such as a special project or course; or it may stem from an informal decision by a group of staff members. Regardless of the impetus, gerontology professionals and agencies must take the responsibility for preparing to work with diverse cultures and ethnic groups.

Building on Previous Recommendations

During the last 15 years much attention has been directed toward ethnicity and mental health. This attention was due largely to the recognition that a majority of mental health centers were not providing culturally sensitive treatment to minority clients. The

1976 White House Conference on Ethnicity and Mental Health was instrumental in making mental health professionals aware of the importance of ethnicity in assisting clients. Later, the President's Commission on Mental Health (1978) developed a set of components to be utilized in training mental health workers to work with ethnic/minority individuals. These components are also relevant for gerontology professionals who are being trained to provide service to the ethnic aged. They include

- the professional's understanding of his/her own ethnic identity and the factors that are obstacles or strengths in his/her ability to understand and communicate with diverse groups of patients;
- awareness of how ethnic traditions shape the attitudes, values, modes of verbal and nonverbal communication, and family structures of patients and of the various groups in the community;
- awareness of how the American experience of immigration, internal migration, and industrialization has further modified these traditions;
- awareness of how these factors need to be taken into account in diagnosis (what is culturally adaptive or maladaptive behavior and what is psychopathological), treatment, and planning of services;
- learning to use the natural support systems of communities and neighborhoods;
- modifying old treatment methods and developing new ones to reach different ethnic groups;
- learning skills in intergroup techniques to work more effectively with various ethnic groups in developing coalitions and reducing group tensions;
- special attention to the unique needs of foreign-born mental health personnel in helping them to better understand and work with diverse ethnic groups.

Basic Principles

The following section is designed as a guide for both the practitioner and the educator interested in planning a training program to deal with the ethnic aged. It is the author's belief that certain basic principles must be introduced into the training program if a particular agency is truly interested in addressing ethnic/minority aging issues.

Broadening the Professionals' Cultural World View

The first task is to increase the professionals' awareness of their own cultural traditions and ethnicity. Emphasis should be placed on how cultural values can enhance or impede work with diverse ethnic groups. During this introductory phase, professionals should be encouraged to identify and become knowledgeable about the ethnic and racial cultures that surround the particular area of service, for example, their heritage, belief systems, attitudes toward receiving assistance, and informal support systems. An awareness of the importance of respect, privacy, dignity, and shame and the specific implications that they have on providing services to the ethnic aged are essential.

Enhancing Culturally Relevant Skills and Programs

How the provider deals with the individual cultural aspects of the client often determines the outcome of the intervention. Professionals need to be sensitized to the cultural appropriateness of such skills as eye contact, body language, tone and speech rate, and nonthreatening topics of conversation. Training needs to center on how an agency can make its services more accessible and acceptable to the ethnic aged. Such strategies as the recruitment of ethnic older adults to act as peer counselors, the development of an outreach program, or a translation service should be explored.

Addressing Resistance

There has been considerable debate about the advisability of establishing separate programs for the ethnic aged. A high percentage of service providers reject the concept of altering or separating services on the ground that the ethnic aged would not welcome it because of their mistrust for the majority population (Holmes, 1983). In addition, many providers feel that their contact with ethnic groups provides them with sufficient knowledge, and they question the need for specialized training. Such issues will invariably surface and must be dealt with in an open, nonconfrontational fashion. One way to engage participation is to invite carefully selected experts to address the entire staff, stimulate enthusiasm, and initiate ongoing seminars on the topic. Also, establishing a safe context in which stereotyping and generalizing about cultural and personal differences can be expressed is essential.

Entering the System Effectively

How a training program is introduced, and the extent to which staff dynamics are assessed can often determine the success or failure of the program. It is essential for the executive director of an agency to establish the priority of the program by committing the needed time, resources, and administrative participation to develop the training sessions adequately. This conveys to the staff a clear message that the agency seriously supports the training initiative and expects workers to participate actively. Efforts should be made to elicit suggestions from certain staff regarding the content of the training sessions to establish a team approach to the subject area.

Selecting Training Participants

In a large agency where the goal is to influence agencywide practices, it is cumbersome and impractical to offer training workshops to everyone. Initially, it is best to select a small group of practitioners who have demonstrated their interest and skill in working with ethnic groups. Intensive training targeted at a core group can generate interest throughout the agency. In addition, a core group can help reduce the intensity of resistance. We must recognize that ethnicity is a highly political and emotional issue that stirs up hidden agendas, existing intergroup conflicts, and positive or negative reactions. A core group of trainers, known to the staff and familiar with agency issues, can be a model of the way to address resistance positively. These individuals can demonstrate the importance of acknowledging differences, exploring fears of being labeled prejudiced or racist, and discussing the consequences of not addressing the difficulties at all.

Taking a Multiethnic Perspective

The point is continually made that the United States is a pluralistic society. A common error in many ethnicity training programs is to focus exclusively on one ethnic group. Important as it may seem to present an in-depth examination of a specific ethnic group, such an approach ignores the reality of pluralism in America. Presenting training in ethnic/minority aging that crosses all racial/ethnic groups has a better chance of attaining its objective because it allows commonalities among diverse groups to be understood. Expanding the existing Area Agency on Aging minority training initiatives to include the Euro-American elderly would satisfy this concern. Certainly, each ethnic group handles issues differently, but research has also demonstrated that the problems faced by the European aged are similar to those of other minority elderly.

Focusing on the Strengths of Ethnicity

A major emphasis of training should be to help participants discover the varied coping mechanisms that grow out of different heritages and traditions, and learn how to mobilize them in service to aged clients. Practitioners need to be conscious of how positive ethnic identity contributes to higher self-esteem. They should be aware of how the family, extended kin network, informal support systems, religious and folk beliefs, and other cultural values can be powerful instruments in helping ethnic aged to cope. However, these positive aspects may be overromanticized or neglected in weighty discussions of the special problems that face each ethnic group. The trainer must set an appropriate climate and guide the group to be more conscious of those ethnic and religious aspects that help individuals see themselves positively and cope with problems on a daily basis.

INTEGRATION OF PRINCIPLES INTO A TRAINING MODEL

The principles outlined above should be utilized as a guide in planning a professional program regarding the ethnic aged. The training objectives of such a program should include (a) an awareness of one's own ethnic and cultural identity, (b) an appreciation of other cultures, (c) development of skills in working with the ethnic aged, (d) brainstorming service and planning interventions on behalf of the ethnic aged.

Below is a suggested outline of topics, activities, and curriculum models for a training program that could be utilized by an Area Agency on Aging, a senior citizens center, or an academic institution. Each module can act as one particular training session or be condensed into a 1-day workshop. However, the curriculum has been designed to build on each subsequent module and follow a specific order. As with any guide or model, it can be adjusted to suit the needs of a particular agency, course, or situation.

Module I: Ethnic Consciousness

Objective

Experiential ethnic sharing—to bring one's ethnic background into conscious thought and see how it relates to behavior and attitudes toward aging.

Content and Process

The trainer should explain to the staff that this is going to be an ethnic sharing experience, and everyone will have a turn to speak. Each participant should be asked to address the following questions:

1. Identify yourself ethnically (Italian American, Black American, Jewish American, half Irish/half Polish, White Anglo-Saxon Protestant, and so forth).
2. Describe the area you lived in while growing up (geographic location, type of neighborhood, and so forth).
3. Discuss your family background. What are the ethnic backgrounds of your parents? Where were they born? What do/did they do? Who are other important family members? How do/did they influence you?
4. Relate one positive and one negative aspect of your ethnic background.
5. What were the attitudes and values toward aging expressed in your family?
6. Define what an *ethnic American* is.

The trainers should begin by sharing their backgrounds as models for the group. They should purposely go into detail and relate appropriate anecdotes. This gives everyone permission to talk about personal stories and feelings. The participant sitting beside the leader speaks next, followed by each person in turn around the circle.

After four or five people have spoken, ask others of the same ethnic background whether their experiences were similar or different. You may want to ask someone how they felt about what they had heard from a member of a background different from their own.

Participants should not be allowed to talk abstractly or give opinions. They must speak about themselves initially and relate personal experiences, anecdotes, and feelings.

Listen carefully for specific ethnic characteristics or ambivalence, and interrupt to ask for elaboration. Probe to clarify and help individuals relate their feelings.

Leave time at the end of the session for staff to process the experience.

Module II: The Worldview of the Ethnic Aged

Objective

To increase participant awareness of the needs and concerns of the ethnic aged.

Content and Process

It is essential that the trainer both address the stereotypes applied to the ethnic aged and foster participants' sensitivity to their world view and feelings.

1. Ask participants to write a 1-page essay about their own perceptions of a specific elderly ethnic group (discussion could include such variables as life-style, leisure activities, economic status, language fluency, and so forth). This activity can be done individually or in small groups. Have participants present each profile to the group and determine the stereotype and erroneous information in each, if any. Utilize existing research to address the validity of each stereotype.
2. Ask each participant to assume he/she is an older ethnic immigrant with limited English language fluency. On another sheet of paper, indicate at least three problems that limited language proficiency creates in old age. Describe the feelings generated by each of these problems.
3. Recruit five or six ethnic older adults from the community

who are willing to address the group. Ask these individuals to react to the discussion generated from the above activity. The trainer should guide the panel in discussing particular concerns about being an ethnic elderly American.

Module III: Skill Development in Working with Ethnic Families

Objective

To increase participants' ability to intervene with ethnic families in crises.

Content and Process

Present a mini-lecture on ethnicity, family, and aging. Concentrate on the importance of family within different ethnic groups. Highlight the particular crisis situations that family members experience in caring for a disabled older parent or spouse. Hand out Mostwin's (1979) summary of different ethnic groups' responses to outsiders:

Czechoslovaks—admit strangers with reservations. The family will ask for services but will remain distant. A standardized approach will be offensive.

Estonians—strangers admitted with great reservation. Asking for help will be delayed. A mental health problem is viewed as degrading. The family is too proud to accept help. The stranger should know the language and facts about Estonia.

Hungarians—prefer not to admit strangers. The family tries to solve problems at home. If they perceive care to be definitely needed, it will be requested, but the stranger should be sensitive to cultural differences.

Poles—reluctant to expose weakness to stranger. The family will not seek help on their own initiative except in an emergency and then reluctantly. The stranger should be respectful, should be introduced by a trusted person, and should be clear about service.

Ukrainians—the family would rather starve than seek help. If in need, they will first consult the priest or a person of Ukrainian background. The stranger should speak the language, be of Slavic background, and be very formal (using Mrs., Miss, or Mr., and never first names).

Lithuanians—fearful and mistrustful of strangers. They will not ask for help. They feel it is a shame to accept charity, and that it is an insult to be offered advice.

Techniques

1. Ask each participant what skills and knowledge would be needed to work with the above-mentioned groups.
2. How could the agency develop a program that would be culturally appropriate in working with these groups?
3. Develop a role-playing situation with the trainer acting as a family member (could be any ethnic group above) who is being interviewed by an agency staff person. Have the group critique the staff person's body language, eye contact, choice of questions, and so forth.
4. As a group, determine the skills that will need further practice and knowledge.

Module IV: Informal Support Systems

Objective

There is evidence that by the time people apply for professional services they have already sought less formal help. They probably have a deep sense of frustration and failure when the lay helping system or quasi-institutional system has not worked for them.

A community profile and/or exercise may be introduced to identify formal and informal systems of support in the communities served by the agency. It would include the demographic and historical development of the subcommunities; the spontaneous and natural support systems—family, neighborhood, self-help and peer groups, informal helpers, and caregivers; organized supports not directed by professionals—social, fraternal, religious, and self-help organizations; and professionally directed agencies and organizations—schools, youth agencies, health, and mental health agencies.

Content and Process

- The profile may be developed by a small study group on the staff.
- Bring in representatives of community groups to talk to the staff.
- Arrange staff trips into the neighborhoods.

• Determine which ethnic groups have strong or weak support
  systems and how they can be strengthened or utilized more
  effectively.

Some questions to be asked include the following:

1. Where and how do people cluster (e.g., street corners, in
   front of houses, bars, vacant lots, shade trees, mini-parks,
   stores, churches, etc.)?
2. What is the population density? How do people respond to
   density as compared with people in your own culture or
   socioeconomic group?
3. What kinds of affect are observed in adults, in children?
4. Which sex and age groups are seen together (e.g., older
   men alone, with older women, with younger men; young
   couples with chaperones, families, etc.)?
5. How do the sexes interact?
6. How do family members interact?
7. Are there many elderly people? With whom do they associate? How are they treated? Do they differ in the above
   respects from other adults?
8. What is the noise level (street noise, music loudness, etc.)
   in your terms and in the culture's terms?
9. What phenomena observed in the neighborhoods might be
   construed as stressors (e.g., lack of air conditioning, fast-
   moving automobiles, broken mailboxes, etc.)?
10. Are they perceived as stressors in the way that your culture
    might perceive them? Are there other possible stressors
    that may not be readily visible but that may be inferred
    from behavior?
11. Observe the neighborhoods in structural terms. Is there
    neighborhood self-containment (e.g., churches, stores,
    laundromats, hardware stores, funeral homes, healers,
    shopping centers)? Are these far away or within easy walk-
    ing distance?
12. How far must people travel to obtain medical or social
    service assistance?
13. What resources might be tapped for emotional and physical
    help or enrichment (examples: healing, recreational, spir-
    itual, educational, interpersonal, economic, etc.)?
14. Are there recreational areas—parks, bowling alleys, dance
    halls, community centers, and so forth?

15. How do you react to the phenomena observed?
16. Examine your own mode of approach and communication patterns with community residents. Did they enhance or detract from your getting to know the people and their environment?

Module V: Identify the Ethnic Issues in Practice

Objective

The trainer should tell the group that the task for this session is to develop a staff consensus on the 10 most pressing practice issues around ethnicity and aging.

The reason to develop a consensus should be explained by the trainer. Without clarity and consensus as to what the important issues are, very little progress can be made to achieve effective solutions.

Content and Process

The leader should ask the group to name the ethnocultural issues that arise in practice. Everything is written on a blackboard without editing, exactly as worded by the participants; alternate wording should be approved by the person who stated the problem. The 10 problems that occur most often in working with the elderly should be read aloud so that everyone will be familiar with them, and they should be ranked according to their seriousness. The five most important problems will be worked on in the next session.

It is important for the trainer to help clarify the problems. For example, very often the Jewish aged in the community use services easily, but Blacks and Italians do not come into the agency. The leader should help the group determine whether the issue is a result of culturally incompatible services or their needs not being met adequately within their own families and/or communities.

PROBLEMS THAT TRAINERS ENCOUNTER

Developing a training program that focuses on ethnicity is not an easy undertaking. We would like to delineate several issues that may arise and offer suggestions that a trainer may utilize in the context of the session. First, it is not unusual when material is presented on a variety of different ethnic groups that some participants will comment, "Aren't you stereotyping?" A strategy in addressing this situation is to state at the beginning of the training session that it is often difficult to talk about different ethnic groups without making some generalizations.

While it is imperative that trainers avoid rigid stereotyping, it is important for practitioners to recognize that members of particular ethnic and religious groups may share distinctive values. Not all Italians have tight family relationships; not all Poles suffer in silence; not all Irish are deeply religious. Italians, however, are probably more like each other than they are like the Irish, the Poles, or other ethnic groups.

Second, as with other topics introduced in a training session, there may be hidden agendas that deflect from the focus of the presentation. For example, the trainer may want to talk about ethnicity, but the staff is interested in discussing staff morale. Group and individual relationships, political and ideological conflicts, and management issues may be some of the hidden agendas that can undermine a training program on ethnicity. It is critical that the trainer be aware that these issues may "lurk" beneath the surface. The trainer must restate the purpose of the training session with the group and not let organizational issues that are outside the realm of ethnicity detract from the stated goals.

Third, ethnic and racial conflicts between agency staff members can jeopardize the outcome of the training session. Sometimes, whether through competition or conflict, professionals from different ethnic and racial groups view the ethnicity training session as an opportunity to air their particular differences. The trainer must be aware of these issues and their history, and who the principal players are, and must help the group separate what can be useful for discussion and learning purposes and what issues should be addressed by the administration in a different context.

Finally, it is possible that some gerontology professionals have had previous exposure to training sessions that have addressed ethnicity. Some of these experiences may not have been positive and may color the outlook of the professional. It is important for the trainer to emphasize that this training experience is different; that is, multiethnic in focus, not simply addressing one group, and based on the positive aspects of ethnicity.

IDENTIFYING RESOURCES FOR TRAINING

An agency interested in developing a training program on the ethnic aged has a variety of resources on which to draw in developing a program. Since many agencies are facing severe budgetary constraints, it may be essential to develop a program that does not require hiring an outside trainer to facilitate the effort. We have attempted to identify community resources and material that can be incorporated and that would not require extensive funds in developing a training program.

The first place to look for resources to assist in developing a training program on the ethnic aged is within the agency itself. Many agencies contain staff persons and volunteers with rich ethnic backgrounds. Too often, professionalism functions to prohibit staff from sharing skills and knowledge about their ethnic backgrounds. Similarly, nonprofessional staff, often more ethnically identified, do not offer their knowledge because the norm of the agency is often to downplay the role of ethnicity. These ethnic staff can be recruited to help in planning a training program, making a presentation, or being a consultant. For example, a nutrition program within an ethnic community may contain a volunteer who has extensive knowledge regarding how to identify and approach Hungarian elderly who need a home-delivered meal. This individual could be utilized as a resource within a training session on developing culturally appropriate outreach efforts.

Many urban communities contain a diverse array of ethnic organizations. Members of these organizations often are professionals with skills in a variety of helping disciplines. Agencies often fail to realize that ethnic organizations can be utilized as a resource in both helping to identify the needs of the ethnic aged and addressing ways to deal with such problems. An agency interested in developing a multiethnic training program could call on a variety of ethnic leaders to make presentations regarding their community's elders.

Another untapped training resource lies within a community's academic institutions. Research on ethnic/minority aging has increased dramatically over the past decade. The knowledge developed through these research efforts could be translated into specific methods of gerontological practice. Agencies should call on these researchers for staff presentations, conferences, and consultation. However, when academics are utilized in this capacity, emphasis should be placed on translating research into practice methods.

Agencies that wish to develop training programs on ethnicity and aging can utilize an extensive amount of material generated from previous efforts. The bibliography on ethnicity and aging compiled by Murguia et al. (1984) contains a variety of citations oriented toward minority training models. Unfortunately, as mentioned previously, little is available regarding the training of gerontology professionals in addressing the needs of the Euro-American elderly. However, some of this material could be adapted easily for this purpose.

In addition, we recommend that gerontologists explore the applicability of training models developed in other fields. For example, the Center on Ethnicity, Behaviour and Communications and the Institute for American Pluralism of the American Jewish Committee have since 1968 conducted training and generated a wide array of publications in the area of ethnicity and mental health. Also, Drs. John Spiegel and John Papajohn of the Florence Heller School, Brandeis University, have been operating training programs on ethnicity. A detailed description of their work is contained in the *Final Report of Training Programs in Ethnicity and Mental Health* (1983).

FUTURE DIRECTIONS

It is imperative that a systematic approach be developed to train professionals in addressing the needs of Euro-American elderly. To date, little has been done on a national basis to upgrade the skills of service providers in working with this group. One possible strategy in addressing this need is the development of a national training resource center. The purpose of such a center would be to provide service professionals and ethnic leaders with information and training on working with Euro-American elderly. Emphasis would be given to translating existing research on the ethnic/minority aged into practice models.

Area Agencies on Aging should be held accountable for training gerontology professionals in serving all ethnic groups within their catchment areas. Yearly evaluations should be conducted that indicate the following:

• frequency of workshops or training sessions for addressing the service needs of the ethnic aged;

- breakdown of the content to indicate the ethnic groups addressed in the sessions;
- involvement of the ethnic aged in both planning the training sessions and delivering presentations;
- assessment of the utilization and underutilization by various European groups of services funded through the Older Americans Act;
- future training efforts to sensitize gerontology professionals regarding ethnocultural factors in service delivery.

CONCLUSION

Training gerontology professionals to address the needs of the Euro-American elderly has been minimal. Existing training programs that address the concerns of the minority aged (Blacks, Hispanics, Asian Americans, and so forth) should be enlarged to include the European aged. Such expansion would provide gerontology professionals with a well-rounded knowledge base in providing services to all ethnic groups.

Many older adult service agencies through the support of Area Agencies on Aging need to provide more opportunities for professional staff to explore the ways in which ethnocultural factors impact on service utilization and provision. In particular, sensitizing staff to their own ethnicity is critical in agencies that are addressing the needs of a wide array of ethnic groups. Failing to address the impact of ethnicity can lead to stereotypical thinking, staff/client conflict, and reduced program impact.

In developing a training program regarding the ethnic aged, various principles need to be incorporated by the trainer into the content presented. Some of the more important principles include sensitizing professionals to the cultural appropriateness of communication styles, utilizing the ethnic aged to present material in order to lower participant resistance, and training a core group of professionals initially to develop a strong agency foundation in the topic area.

The training model presented can be adapted easily based on the needs of the participants and those of the agency. Undoubtedly, the success of ethnicity training is dependent largely on the trainer's ability to identify possible hidden agendas and to keep the group focused on the goal of the training session.

13

Serving the Needs of Euro-American Elderly through Research

David Guttmann, D.S.W.

Once the preacher of Zlotchov, a small town in eastern Galicia, was asked how we are to understand that we could do what our fathers did. He expounded:

> Just as our fathers found new ways of serving, each a new service according to his character: one the service of love, the other that of stern justice, the third that of beauty, so each one of us in his own way shall devise something new in the light of teachings and of service, and do what has not yet been done. (Buber, 1976, p. 3)

Despite a growing body of literature on aging, research about minority aged in general and about Euro-American elderly in particular, has received scant attention by gerontologists. Of the 44 works reviewed by Murguia et al. (1984), the majority concentrate on four ethnic groups among American elderly: Italian, Jewish, Polish, and Slavic. Moreover, the few studies listed as *comparative of White ethnics* include the same ethnic groups.

Whereas there is detailed literature on the racial minorities—Black, Hispanic, Asian-Pacific, and Native Americans—under many subheadings such as demographic and socioeconomic characteristics; health, medicine, and folk medicine; housing; education; leisure, marriage, and family; social participation and support services, the paucity of studies on Euro-American elderly did not warrant similar listing by the authors of *Ethnicity and Aging: A Bibliography* (Murguia et al., 1984).

An even more serious shortcoming in this bibliography is the fact that the variations found in ethnic groups are simply ignored. Yet there can be no serious discussion on Euro-American elderly from a sociocultural perspective without reference to those distinctions. A religioethnic group is distinguished from other ethnic groups by the significance of religion in the social organization of the lives of its members. On the other hand, nationality-based ethnic groups such as Hungarians, Greeks, Latvians, Lithuanians, and others define themselves chiefly by national origin, ethnic language, and tradition (Watson, 1982).

At least Murguia et al. (1984) have provided some evidence to the existence of Euro-American elderly as distinct from other minority groups. Other authors of well-known textbooks on aging (Butler & Lewis, 1982; Crandall, 1980; Huyck & Hoyer, 1982; Kart, 1985; Schaie & Geiwitz, 1982) with the exception of Watson (1982) avoided the subject altogether. Even authorities such as Atchley (1985) and Lowy (1985) failed to mention Euro-American elderly among the ethnic/minority groups.

Such lack of recognition, while not condoned, could have been understood prior to the 1981 White House Conference on Aging and the 1980 hearings of the Commission on Civil Rights. However, once these two governmental forums had legitimized the existence of Euro-American elderly as a cultural/ethnic minority, the omission of these people in textbooks used extensively in colleges and universities for teaching social gerontology is an "insult of ignorance."

In this chapter an attempt will be made to review and list areas in which there are recognized gaps in research about serving the needs of elderly Euro-Americans. The term *research* will be used here as an endeavor aimed at discovering, substantiating, and assessing, on the one hand, the needs of Euro-American elderly for services and, on the other hand, the capabilities of ethnic communities to provide the needed supports to their own elderly members.

Since the focus of this chapter is on research related to service provision and service utilization, no attempt will be made to deal with methodological issues. Those who are interested in this aspect of research are advised to consult the works of several well-known researchers and authors in the field of minority aging (Cuellar, Stanford, & Miller-Soule, 1982; Stanford, 1979).

IDENTIFIED GAPS IN KNOWLEDGE ABOUT EURO-AMERICAN ELDERLY

The study completed by this author and his associates during 1977–1979 (Guttmann et al., 1979b) serves as the basis for the identification of gaps in research about Euro-American elderly. This study was the first to highlight the situation of the white ethnic aged in eight different cultural groups, and it has served many researchers as baseline data about the Euro-American elderly. For more detailed information concerning this study and its findings, see the article by Guttmann et al. (1979b) in *Ethnicity and Aging.*

On the basis of these and other research findings concerning Euro-American elderly, identified gaps in research about this segment of the aged population fall into four areas:

1. acquisition of basic knowledge about the conditions and the needs of Euro-American elderly in specific ethnic groups;
2. ways and means in which ethnic communities can meet the needs of Euro-American elderly;
3. ways in which the government and other formal support systems can assist ethnic communities to offer culturally relevant services to the Euro-American elderly who need such services;
4. issues of *adequate criteria* by which services are measured.

These four categories encompass many aspects of life in which our present knowledge is minuscule: family structure, social support networks, environmental conditions, attitudes, personality traits, health care practices, coping behavior, and so forth. Yet we know that a combination of these factors influences the quality of life in old age and the process of aging. These four areas will comprise, therefore, the bulk of this chapter.

Researching the Needs of Euro-American Elderly

In researching the needs of Euro-American elderly for services, we have to begin with a definition of the term *needs.* A need, as opposed to a wish, indicates a lack of something requisite, desirable, or useful (Webster, 1978), or a condition requiring supply or relief. *Need* also means to be in want of the means of subsistence or to be under obligation or necessity. The most obvious need, which is recognized by researchers, policymakers, ethnic community leaders, and service providers alike, is for basic information about Euro-American elderly. This means intensive data collection with regard to the socioeconomic and demographic characteristics of the elderly in the many ethnic groups designated as Euro-American.

One of the means by which this research objective can be met is to require the U.S. Census Bureau to include additional items in its questionnaires about the ethnic background of older Americans, including a determination whether we are dealing with old or new immigrants, or with natives (those who were born in the United States but still identify themselves as Euro-American). General surveys that ignore such differences can no longer be considered appropriate and relevant for providing accurate and useful information in planning policies and services for a heterogeneous body of consumers.

The U.S. Census Bureau is not the only resource for this purpose, however. Euro-American ethnic organizations that represent various groups at the national, regional, or local levels can undertake a needs assessment survey of their members over 65 years of age to learn about their conditions and needs for services.

Another area for useful research concerning the needs of Euro-American elderly is related to discovering the truly needy among the residents of the ethnic community. It is a well-known fact that many Euro-American elderly do not admit the necessity for services because of cultural attitudes against receiving and using public benefits. Research designed to deal with problems could separate and document those cases that require basic survival services from those that need emotional or social supports. At the present, research related to the living conditions of millions of ethnic elderly is minimal. In one study (Guttmann et al., 1979b) 20% of the elderly respondents admitted a need for one or more basic services of income, housing, health care, and so forth; yet the majority of these people did not utilize available services. We need greater understanding of the factors that are operating in such situations, especially insight into the realities of ethnic communities and the dynamics of neighborhood life as well as an understanding of perceptions of people regarding life in ethnic communities.

It is also necessary to replicate former studies of needs assessments for Euro-American elderly in order to learn whether over time their living conditions have changed for better or for worse. For example, in the study cited above, one out of five retired men and two out of five retired women reported that they had no one to whom to turn for help when they had basic needs. Deprived of life-sustaining social networks and interaction with neighbors or ethnic or public organizations, their aloneness may lead to increasingly aberrant behavior and serious mental health impairments.

Research aimed at discovering needs of Euro-American elderly for public and/or private services cannot be complete without studying the meanings that each cultural group attaches to such terms as *needs, resources,* and *use of services.* These meanings usually differ from one ethnic group to another and from one social class to another within the ethnic group. Research that does not take such differences into consideration can result in a biased or distorted picture of its subjects. The realization of prevailing cultural diversity in perceptions, attitudes, and behavior of people, as pointed out in a previous chapter, necessitates studying basic problems in each ethnic group.

Researching Ways and Means of Meeting the Needs of the Euro-American Elderly

A notorious shortcoming of many studies about ethnicity, minorities, and Euro-American elderly in general is the lack of data about the strengths of ethnic communities that can be taken into consideration in addressing the needs of Euro-American elderly for communal services. Ethnic communities differ from each other in service provisions to the elderly, not only in attitudes and available resources but also in the extent to which they perceive their own strengths that can be marshalled in solving individual and group problems. For example, the Jewish community (Guttmann et al., 1979b) has a well-developed network of health care services such as hospitals, mental health facilities, nursing homes, group and boarding homes, visiting nurse services, and homemaking/ home health aid services (see Tables 13.1 and 13.2). This same ethnic group has also developed a variety of services in housing and financial assistance as well as transportation services.

There are known historical/cultural traditions and attitudes in operation with respect to the ways in which ethnic groups organize their available strengths and resources for meeting the needs of their elderly. While the Jewish community over the centuries has refined its organized response to the Biblical commandment to "Honor thy father and thy mother," other ethnic

TABLE 13.1. Institutional Supports: Organized Services in Ethnic Community (Percentages) ($N = 180$)

Ethnic Group	Does Your Community Have These Services?			Nature of financial assistance			What kind of organized transportation?			
	Housing	Future Housing Plans	Financial Assistance	Community and Fraternity	Other Family	Transportation	Formal	Informal	Other	Unspecified
Estonian	5.0	20.0	25.0	5.0	5.0	10.0	0.0	45.0	0.0	55.0
Latvian	0.0	20.0	40.0	0.0	0.0	30.0	10.0	40.0	0.0	50.0
Lithuanian	0.0	15.0	25.0	15.0	5.0	10.0	5.0	35.0	0.0	60.0
Greek	0.0	50.0	80.0	0.0	0.0	5.0	0.0	80.0	0.0	5.0
Italian	10.0	30.0	5.0	5.0	0.0	10.0	0.0	15.0	15.0	60.0
Jewish	90.0	80.0	85.0	55.0	5.0	100.	90.0	0.0	25.0	10.0
Hungarian	0.0	5.0	30.0	20.0	5.0	0.0	0.0	35.0	0.0	60.0
Polish (Washington)	0.0	10.0	40.0	25.0	5.0	30.0	20.0	20.0	25.0	35.0
Polish (Baltimore)	5.0	10.0	15.0	0.0	5.0	0.0	10.0	60.0	30.0	0.0
Total sample	12.2	26.7	38.3	13.9	3.3	21.7	15.0	36.7	11.1	37.2

From D. Guttmann et al., *Informal and Formal Support Systems and their Effect on the Lives of the Elderly in Selected Ethnic Groups* (Appendix, Section D, Table 16). The National Catholic School of Social Service, The Catholic University of America, 1979.

TABLE 13.2 Institutional Supports: Organized Services in Ethnic Community (Percentages) $N = 180$

Ethnic Group	Safety	Group Action	Social Service Agency	Central Referral	Effectiveness of information and referral service		
					Effective	Moderately Effective	Unspecified
Estonian	5.0	5.0	10.0	25.0	30.0	0.0	70.0
Latvian	0.0	25.0	30.0	30.0	30.0	5.0	65.0
Lithuanian	0.0	35.0	5.0	15.0	5.0	5.0	90.0
Greek	5.0	60.0	30.0	65.0	65.0	5.0	30.0
Italian	10.0	50.0	15.0	20.0	30.0	15.0	55.0
Jewish	10.0	100.0	95.0	100.0	70.0	25.0	5.0
Hungarian	0.0	25.0	15.0	15.0	15.0	0.0	85.0
Polish (Washington)	0.0	25.0	20.0	10.0	5.0	15.0	80.0
Polish (Baltimore)	5.0	70.0	20.0	15.0	5.0	20.0	75.0
Total Sample	3.9	43.9	26.7	32.8	28.3	10.1	61.7

From D. Guttmann et al., *Informal and Formal Support Systems and their Effect on the Lives of the Elderly in Selected Ethnic Groups* (Appendix, Section D, Table 16). The National Catholic School of Social Service, The Catholic University of America, 1979.

groups used different means to activate their own response to this commandment. In crisis situations and on an individual basis, each of the eight ethnic groups included in the study cited above provided some sort of relief to needy elderly, but in very different degrees (See Table 13.3).

Research, therefore, is needed to learn more about those ethnic groups that so far have escaped the attention of researchers as to the ways they meet the needs of their elderly members. We need to learn much more about the helping networks to which the elderly may turn in the ethnic community. We need to learn more about the capabilities of these support networks to respond to various needs and about the ways in which ethnic community strengths and resources can be combined with other public supports for assisting the Euro-American elderly in need. Such research would create new awareness about the ethnic community and neighborhood as a critical resource to maintain, nurture, develop, and enhance physical, mental, spiritual, and social health in aging. Such research could be beneficial to the ethnic community as well since it would help in discovering hidden strengths that may be utilized. This would not only benefit the Euro-American elderly but also would help prevent the disintegration of the ethnic family and the community along with their distinct culture, institutions, and life-styles.

Another important area for research relates to religion and aging. We know that a significant strength and resource of the ethnic community is vested in the ethnic churches/synagogues and the clergy. Organized religion plays an important role in the lives of many ethnic elderly because it is an intrinsic part of their cultural identity (see Chapter 7, "Religion and the Church"). Until recently, little attention was paid to the centrality of the spiritual dimension in old age. Like its complex counterpart, ethnicity, religion is another aspect of culture and civilization that dwells within the human heart. We may be able to classify, measure, analyze, and interpret its outward expressions, but who can fathom its inward dimensions? No wonder that most published research on religion and aging deals with religious practices, or lack of them, in institutionalized ways.

Fecher, who compiled an excellent *Bibliography on Religion and Aging* (1982), admits that most attempts at scholarly studies on inward, personal religion have been spotty, inconclusive, and even contradictory, and that the real work remains to be done. This is, then, an area that waits to be addressed by researchers in aging.

TABLE 13.3 Institutional Supports: Community Provision of Housing for Elderly in Times of Crisis (Percentages) $N = 180$

Ethnic Group	In Crisis, Does Community Provide Housing for Elderly? If so, in what way?					
	yes	Formal Support	Informal Support	Combination of Formal & Informal	Other	Unspecified Response
Estonian	70.0	35.0	15.0	5.0	10.0	35.0
Latvian	60.0	25.0	0.0	10.0	30.0	35.0
Lithuanian	50.0	20.0	5.0	0.0	5.0	70.0
Greek	55.0	0.0	10.0	20.0	30.0	40.0
Italian	35.0	10.0	25.0	5.0	0.0	60.0
Jewish	85.0	55.0	0.0	15.0	20.0	10.0
Hungarian	50.0	15.0	20.0	5.0	5.0	55.0
Polish (Washington)	25.0	15.0	10.0	0.0	5.0	65.0
Polish (Baltimore)	15.0	0.0	5.0	0.0	15.0	80.0
Total Sample	49.4	19.5	10.0	6.7	13.4	50.1

From D. Guttmann et al, *Informal and Formal Support Systems and their Effect on the Lives of the Elderly in Selected Ethnic Groups* (Appendix, Section D, Table 20). The National Catholic School of Social Service, The Catholic University of America, 1979.

A review of the various support services provided by the church such as financial assistance; burial services; social, recreational, and nutritional services; and transportation for needy elderly revealed wide fluctuations from one ethnic group to another (Guttmann et al., 1979b). Similar findings were reported by these subjects with respect to the services provided by the clergy such as visiting the sick, counseling, and giving spiritual support.

We need to know to what extent these findings are representative and applicable not only to the eight ethnic communities involved in that study but in other ethnic communities where Euro-American elderly live. We need to learn more about those projects, techniques, and efforts that ethnic churches and their clergy exert in meeting the needs of the elderly—whether alone or in combination with other communal service providers (see Tables 13.4, 13.5, and 13.6).

Researching the Need for Culturally Relevant Services to Euro-American Elderly

A far-reaching idea for the helping professions and providers of services to Euro-American elderly is implied in the term *culturally relevant services.* First coined by the Task Panel on Community Support Systems in the President's Commission on Mental Health (1978), the term refers to services based on the values and norms of a given culture. It reaffirms not only the existence of ethnic groups within the total population, but also requires recognition of ethnocultural differences among the clients by government-sponsored agencies and services. For example, in Guttmann et al.'s (1979b) study nearly half of the respondents had a clear preference for government-provided services, while 25% did not indicate a preference between government and other community or ethnic service providers. Although we have no data on the preferences of the missing 26% of the respondents, the differences were striking in attitude to service provision among the eight ethnic groups of Euro-American elderly that were studied: Greek elderly indicated a preference for government-offered services at more than twice the rate of the Jewish group; Italians, on the other hand, did not like the idea of differentiation between government and nongovernment service provision.

In researching the need for culturally relevant services, attention should be directed to the involvement of social supports and natural helping networks in the overall well-being of the elderly in

TABLE 13.4 Institutional Supports: Services Provided by the Church (Percentages) ($N = 180$)

Ethnic Group	Spiritual	Financial Assistance	Burial	Social Recreation	Nutritional	Organized Transportation	Combination	N.R. D.K.
Estonian	30.0	0.0	0.0	0.0	0.0	0.0	15.0	55.0
Latvian	0.0	5.0	5.0	15.0	0.0	0.0	25.0	50.0
Lithuanian	25.0	0.0	0.0	5.0	0.0	0.0	15.0	55.0
Greek	0.0	0.0	0.0	25.0	0.0	0.0	35.0	40.0
Italian	5.0	0.0	0.0	0.0	10.0	0.0	15.0	70.0
Jewish	0.0	0.0	0.0	30.0	0.0	0.0	65.0	5.0
Hungarian	35.0	0.0	0.0	10.0	0.0	0.0	15.0	40.0
Polish (Washington)	45.0	0.0	0.0	5.0	0.0	10.0	25.0	15.0
Polish (Baltimore)	0.0	0.0	0.0	30.0	0.0	0.0	25.0	45.0
Total Sample	15.6	0.6	0.6	13.3	1.1	1.1	26.1	41.7

From D. Guttmann et al., *Informal and Formal Support Systems and their Effect on the Lives of the Elderly in Selected Ethnic Groups* (Appendix, Section D, Table 21). The National Catholic School of Social Service, The Catholic University of America, 1979.

TABLE 13.5 Institutional Supports: Services Provided by the Clergy (Percentages) (N = 180)

Ethnic Group	Visit sick	Counsel	Spiritual	Other & Comb.	None	N.R./D.K.
Estonian	60.0	0.0	10.0	25.0	5.0	0.0
Latvian	55.0	0.0	5.0	35.0	0.0	5.0
Lithuanian	30.0	0.0	10.0	45.0	5.0	10.0
Greek	10.0	0.0	0.0	90.0	0.0	0.0
Italian	20.0	0.0	5.0	35.0	25.0	15.0
Jewish	5.0	0.0	0.0	50.0	35.0	10.0
Hungarian	15.0	0.0	20.0	30.0	30.0	5.0
Polish	20.0	10.0	10.0	30.0	30.0	5.0
(Washington)						
Polish	55.0	0.0	5.0	30.0	5.0	5.0
(Baltimore)						
Total Sample	30.0	1.1	7.2	42.8	12.8	6.1

From D. Guttmann et al., *Informal and Formal Support Systems and their Effect on the Lives of the Elderly in Selected Ethnic Groups* (Appendix, Section D, Table 21). The National Catholic School of Social Service, The Catholic University of America, 1979.

TABLE 13.6 Institutional Supports: Activities Used Exclusively by Elderly (Percentages) (N = 180)

Ethnic Group	Are there activities used exclusively by elderly?			Why not?			
	Yes	No	No Need	Elderly Included	Community Too Small	Other	Unspecified Response
Estonian	5.0	95.0	0.0	45.0	15.0	20.0	20.0
Latvian	20.0	80.0	5.0	55.0	10.0	5.0	25.0
Lithuanian	10.0	90.0	0.0	50.0	10.0	15.0	25.0
Greek	15.0	85.0	0.0	40.0	0.0	15.0	45.0
Italian	35.0	65.0	10.0	25.0	0.0	5.0	60.0
Jewish	85.0	15.0	0.0	0.0	0.0	0.0	100.
Hungarian	25.0	75.0	0.0	50.0	0.0	10.0	40.0
Polish (Washington)	10.0	90.0	0.0	40.0	10.0	25.0	20.0
Polish (Baltimore)	35.0	65.0	0.0	30.0	0.0	15.0	55.0
Total Sample	26.7	73.3	1.7	37.2	5.0	12.2	43.9

From D. Guttmann et al., *Informal and Formal Support Systems and their Effect on the Lives of the Elderly in Selected Ethnic Groups* (Appendix, Section D, Table 22), The National Catholic School of Social Service, The Catholic University of America, 1979.

ethnic communities. At issue is the need for research that would provide reliable data at the national level on the contributions of these supports to the mental and physical health of Euro-American elderly. Implied in the concept of culturally relevant services are several closely connected factors:

1. recognition of those networks to which people belong and on which they depend: families, friends, neighborhood social networks, work, religious bodies, self-help groups, and other voluntary associations based on principles of intimacy and mutual aid;
2. formal caregiving institutions, their strengths, and potentials;
3. the system of linkages between the natural helping networks and the formal sources of support including the professionals who staff agencies and institutions;
4. the mechanisms used to inform the public on the functions of the above networks and systems (President's Commission on Mental Health, 1978).

Common to all community support systems—self-help, mutual-aid groups, and peer-oriented, helping networks—is the premise that they build on resources already present in the community and that they can provide additional services to supplement those of the government already in existence.

The President's Commission (1978) cautions the reader that their conclusions should not be viewed as a panacea for all problems. What is missing in this list of the many positive functions that community support systems can perform is substantiation. Despite new publications on social support networks and social services (Biegel & Naparstek, 1982; Huttman, 1985; Sauer & Coward, 1985), there is very little reliable research to support the above claims.

There is need for research to separate the myth from the reality of the capacities of support networks to offer culturally relevant services to the Euro-American elderly. For example, can these networks mitigate feelings of loneliness, isolation, and low morale that still plague significant proportions of the elderly (Harris & Associates, 1975; Sussman, 1979)? Can social support networks compensate for losses such as involuntary retirement and widowhood? Can social support networks create a new frame of reference or a new social world peopled with significant others? For whom? Under what conditions? What factors in this creation of

new ties would be culturally relevant? What services will people
need for successful reorientation into the life of the community?

A natural conclusion from the fact that ethnic cultures and
groups exhibit a large degree of variation would be that the
elderly would also differ in the types of networks to which they
want to relate—those that enhance, rather than disrupt their ties
to their accustomed ways of life. For example, Cantor (1979)
found greater degrees of dependence on the locality or neighborhood for friendship and social ties by working-class elderly than by
middle-class elderly. Is this finding generalizable to many Euro-
American elderly or just to those who were included in her
sample?

Another interesting area for study involves the question of
which of the theoretically available informal or natural support
networks is being sought out by service providers, and for what
specific purpose in the attempt to provide culturally relevant
services for a Greek or Polish elderly woman or man who needs
assistance for maintaining independent living in the community?
Finally, what constitutes support according to the subjective perceptions of the recipients?

A generally accepted maxim regarding the elderly Euro-
Americans is that the family remains a bastion of strength and
stability in the ethnic community. Yet, concern about the increased movement of the elderly from the city to the suburbs to
be closer to their families and children has prompted the Administration on Aging of the federal government to issue requests for
research proposals concerning the problems involved in planning
and service delivery of an aging suburbia (Federal Register, September 4, 1985).

Kolm (1980) has characterized eastern and southern Euro-
Americans as people with a strong emphasis on family and community life. Naturally, many other Euro-American elderly ethnic
groups as well as racial minority (and even majority groups) could
make similar claims. There is sufficient research evidence to show
the central importance of family and community for the well-
being of older people in general, including the Euro-American
elderly. Families provide approximately 88% of all home-based
care for frail, functionally deficient or limited elderly who need
such care (Comptroller General, 1977a; National Center for
Health Statistics, 1972).

Moreover, Kulys and Tobin (1980) found that the immediate
family (spouses and children) constitute the most significant persons in the lives of the elderly and that, in case of need, they are

the ones to whom the elderly turn first for assistance. Relatives, friends, and neighbors are the back-up system. Access to support by the family is a significant factor in reducing premature institutionalization and even mortality (Berkman, 1979).

What is missing from this impressive list of culturally relevant services provided by the family to older members is research that would demonstrate a recognition by the formal networks of the skills and dedication that ethnic families exhibit in maintaining the health of older people. We often hear about the sacrifices that adult children make for keeping frail parents at home and about the price they pay in terms of their mental health, but there is little reliable documentation on this subject. There is a lack of research to demonstrate whether attempts by the formal networks of support to assist adult children who care for elderly parents are adequate, relevant, useful, and timely. Nor do we know the impact of the formal services on the quality and quantity of care provided by the natural or informal family network of support. Will such involvement lead to an increase in service utilization by family, or will such assistance be rejected as an intrusion in family affairs?

Researching Adequate Criteria in Service Provision

One of the most frequently cited problems in research on service provision to the elderly is related to the measurement of adequate services. What constitutes this problem was recognized long ago by Rosow (1967), perhaps somewhat cynically or perhaps in earnest, when he stated that the problems of old age are of two general kinds: those that older people actually have and those that experts think they have.

There is no substitute for the subjective approach, in addition to the objective one, to find out what the Euro-American elderly need. There is no substitute for the direct words used by the elderly themselves in expressing concerns about any area of life. Sterne, Phillips, and Rabushka (1974), who studied the situation of the urban elderly poor in the 1970s, point out:

> By allowing each citizen to express his (her) personal, subjective, social wants, i.e. preferences, we arrive at our first and perhaps most important result. As to the white elderly poor they are clearly saying: (1) leave us alone; (2) we are self-reliant and neither need nor want your help; (3) the last two decades have brought about the evolution of an environment in which it is no longer safe to live. We want, in short, the restoration of our neighborhood and way of life to mirror that of an era long since past. (pp. 85–86).

This listing of wants or needs illustrates the difficulties involved in subjective, versus objective, criteria in measuring services. Sterne and others (1974), despite their obvious emphasis on the subjective, have themselves engaged in generalizations based on objective measures in obtaining their data. The designation of White denies the most important subjective fact for Euro-American elderly, their ethnic–cultural identity. There is also a need to study these findings once again, and this time with a more ethnically detailed sample, to learn whether those findings are still applicable to the circumstances of life in the 1980s.

More than 30 years ago the noted educator in social work, Charlotte Towle (1952) maintained that all needs take on different meanings at different stages under different circumstances. For example, if one's sense of self-worth has been consistently maintained through achievement, one's security will be threatened in old age when the means for such needs satisfaction are no longer available. Perhaps a more relevant way (than that listed by Rosow or Sterne and others) to find adequate criteria in service provision research for Euro-American elderly would be to begin by listing what are perceived as common human needs in old age, and for research to concentrate on the corresponding response by service providers to meet those needs.

According to Clark (1967) they are as follows:

- sufficient autonomy to permit continued integrity of the self;
- agreeable relationships with other people, some of whom are willing to provide help when needed without losing respect for the recipient;
- a reasonable amount of personal comfort in body, mind, and physical environment;
- stimulation of the mind and imagination in ways that are not overtaxing of physical health and strength;
- sufficient movement to permit variety in the surroundings;
- some degree of passionate involvement with life, to escape preoccupation with death.

In researching the question as to whether these needs are indeed similar among Euro-American elderly in the many different religious and nationality-based groups, we may arrive at either substantiation or refutation of the above. In either case we will learn more about the perceptions of the elderly as to what really constitutes their needs. We will also learn how these various needs are expressed in each group separately as well as together, in case we deal with more than one ethnic group. We will involve people directly in the process of letting them tell us what they consider important, rather than our telling them. As one of the participants in the U.S. Civil Rights Commission Hearings (1979) on Euro-American elderly said, "Very seldom are the people in the neighborhood who become recipients of whatever programs may be, or the results of action, being talked to. Very seldom do they have an opportunity to be able to have their say" (Testimony of Peter Ujvagi, 1979). The importance of the way research is constructed at the very beginning becomes critical in terms of the kinds of policy actions that ultimately become the end products.

There are many objective, scientific tools currently available to gerontologists for measuring needs, mental health, adjustment to living arrangements, the daily functioning of the elderly, and many other issues both in the community and in various institutions. Those interested in this matter should benefit from the recently published book on this subject by Kane and Kane (1982). By providing detailed information on the various measures—their validity, reliability, and usefulness in conducting research in aging—these authors have enriched our knowledge of the objective aspects of assessment in old age.

However, objective measures usually deal with quantifiable matters and provide only one side of the coin. The other side, the subjective—the more personal, emotional, and much less applicable to scientific measurement—defies measurement. How do people actually feel about a service? Could they express their needs? Were they understood correctly? Was there genuine rapport between them and the service provider, researcher, or interviewer? Were they consulted, truly appreciated, respected, and dealt with decently? All of these feelings, which do not easily translate into measurable quantities and to which no computer card numbers can be assigned, are the ones that constitute adequate services for all people, including Euro-American elderly.

The challenge for researchers in this field of gerontology is to develop, along with the recipients of services, agreed-on criteria by which they may work together in attempting to measure people's perceptions of services. It is relatively easy to measure how many times an elderly person attended a hot-lunch program, but it is much more difficult to assess his/her true feeling about being the recipient of this service; about the attitude of the staff; about the food, the service, and the atmosphere; or the social world of the nutrition program as a whole. It is much more difficult to assess whether the values of independence, self-esteem, and dignity in old age are upheld by the program.

CONCLUSION

This chapter has reviewed four areas of research about Euro-American elderly in which this author has indicated that there are gaps in knowledge: (a) the needs of the Euro-American elderly, (b) ways and means of meeting these needs, (c) culturally relevant services to the Euro-American elderly, and (d) the question of adequate criteria in service provision. Recommendations were also given for future research in each of these areas.

As we look toward the future, we cannot fail to note the hopefulness in the situation of the Euro-American elderly. Despite the apprehension among certain policymakers about the expected growth of the aging population, despite the anticipated burden on the younger generation and on the national budget in caring for the fast-growing segment of the frail and functionally impaired among the elderly, despite future struggles to maintain and improve hard-won benefits; overall, the Euro-American elderly will be party to many hopeful changes and developments already set in motion with regard to the aged population of this country. Euro-American elderly, like their counterparts in both the majority and minority groups of elderly, will be a better educated, more sophisticated group of consumers of services to the aged. They will assume a more active role in national policies and decision-making on their own behalf. This, in turn, will compel researchers and service providers to learn more in depth the kinds of services, service delivery procedures, and methodologies that are best suited to the Euro-American elderly way of life, values, and cultures.

However, until this perhaps utopian outcome can be achieved, there is ample opportunity for researchers who are interested in studying the situation of the Euro-American elderly. There is a need to study factors conducive to activity and involvement in community affairs as well as factors that lead to withdrawal and social isolation among Euro-American elderly. Special efforts need to be directed to identify the unaffiliated elderly and those who lack informal support.

Research is needed to provide data on the mental health needs of the Euro-American aged. There is also a need for more systematic data on the role and importance of ethnic communities as resources in meeting the needs of the ethnic aged. Findings from such research would provide not only a better informational base on the well-being, vulnerability, and service needs of Euro-American elderly, it would also highlight the resources available and the willingness and capabilities of ethnic communities to play various roles in meeting the service needs of Euro-American elderly.

Review of service use and ethnicity research indicates that there is a need for more comprehensive conceptual approaches in applied research on the service needs of the Euro-American elderly. Conceptual frameworks need to systematically conceptualize and operationalize variables on the Euro-American elderly themselves, along with the nature and type of resources available to them, including variables related to service use.

Conceptualization of the Euro-American elderly should include their demographic and socioeconomic status, degree of ethnic identity, ethnic affiliation and practices, health and functional status, social and personal resources, and personal security. The inclusion of these variables will allow a systematic assessment of well-being and vulnerability among Euro-American elderly.

References

Abramson, H. J. (1980). Assimilation and pluralism. In S. T. Thernstrom, A. Orlov, & O. Handlin (Eds.), *Harvard encyclopedia of American ethnic groups* (pp. 150–160). Cambridge, MA: Belknap Press of Harvard University Press.

Administration on Aging. (1979). *Older Americans Act of 1965,* as amended. P.L. 95-178. Washington, DC: U.S. Department of Health, Education, and Welfare.

Alba, R., & Kessler, R. (1979). Patterns of interethnic marriage among American Catholics. *Social Forces, 57,* 1124–1140.

Albanians. (1980). In S. T. Thernstrom, A. Orlov, & O. Handlin (Eds.), *Harvard encyclopedia of American ethnic groups* (pp. 23–28). Cambridge, MA: Belknap Press of Harvard University Press.

Ališauskas, A. (1980). Lithuanians. In S. T. Thernstrom, A. Orlov, & O. Handlin (Eds.), *Harvard encyclopedia of American ethnic groups* (pp. 665–676). Cambridge, MA: Belknap Press of Harvard University Press.

Alonso, W., & Starr, P. (1985, Summer). A nation of numbers watchers. *The Wilson Quarterly,* 103 ff.

Anderson, N., Patten, S., & Greenburg, J. (1980). *A comparison of home care and nursing home care for older persons in Minnesota* (Vol. 3). Minneapolis: University of Minnesota, Hubert H. Humphrey Institute of Public Affairs and Center for Health Services Research.

Antonowsky, A. (1979). *Health, stress and coping.* San Francisco: Jossey-Bass.

Applied Management Sciences. (1975). A study of State Agencies on Aging. [Prepared for Administration on Aging]. Silver Spring, MD: Author.

Arling, G. (1976). The elderly widow: Her family and friends. *Journal of Marriage and the Family, 38,* 737–768.

Atchley, R. (1985). *Social forces in aging* (4th ed.). Belmont, CA: Wadsworth.

Banfield, E. (1958). *The moral basis of a backward society.* Glencoe, IL: Free Press.

Banks, J. A. (1984). *Teaching strategies for ethnic studies* (3rd ed.). Boston: Allen & Bacon.

Bechill, W. (1979). Politics of aging and ethnicity. In D. E. Gelfand & A. J. Kutzik (Eds.), *Ethnicity and aging: Theory, research, and policy* (pp. 137–148). New York: Springer.

Bell, D., Kasschau, P., & Zellman, G. (1976). *Characteristics of the black elderly.* Santa Monica, CA: Rand.

Bengtson, V. L. (1979). Ethnicity and aging: Problems and issues in current social science inquiry. In D. E. Gelfand & A. J. Kutzik (Eds.), *Ethnicity and aging: Theory, research, and policy* (pp. 9–31). New York: Springer.

Benkart, P. (1980). Hungarians. In S. T. Thernstrom, A. Orlov, & O. Handlin (Eds.), *Harvard encyclopedia of American ethnic groups* (pp. 462–471). Cambridge, MA: Belknap Press of Harvard University Press.

Berger, P., & Neuhaus, R. (1977). *To empower people: The role of mediating institutions.* Washington, DC: American Enterprise Institution for Public Policy Research.

Berkman, L. F. (1979, November). *Social networks and physical health: How do we measure the important factors?* Paper presented at the 32nd Annual Scientific Meeting of the Gerontological Society of America, Washington, DC.

Biddle, E. (1981). The American Catholic Irish family. In C. Mindel & R. Habenstein (Eds.), *Ethnic families in America* (pp. 86–114). New York: Elsevier.

Biegel, D. E., Naparstek, A. J., & Khan, M. (1982). *Community support systems and mental health.* New York: Springer.

Biegel, D. E., & Sherman, W. R. (1979). Neighborhood capacity building and the ethnic aged. In D. Gelfand & A. J. Kutzik (Eds.), *Ethnicity and aging: Theory, research & policy* (pp. 320–339). New York: Springer.

Bild, B. R., & Havighurst, R. J. (1976). Senior citizens in great cities: The case of Chicago. *The Gerontologist, 16,* 1–88.

Blessing, P. (1980). Irish. In S. T. Thernstrom, A. Orlov, & O. Handlin (Eds.), *Harvard encyclopedia of American ethnic groups* (pp. 524–545). Cambridge, MA: Belknap Press of Harvard University Press.

Bobango, G. (1980). Romanians. In S. T. Thernstrom, A. Orlov, & O. Handlin (Eds.), *Harvard encyclopedia of American ethnic groups* (pp. 879–885). Cambridge, MA: Belknap Press of Harvard University Press.

Bonutti, K. (1974). *Selected ethnic communities of Cleveland: A socioeconomic study.* Cleveland, OH: Cleveland State University.

Branch, L. G. (1978). *Boston elders.* Program Report. Boston: University of Massachusetts Center for Survey Research.

Brody, E. (1977). *Long-term care for older people.* New York: Human Sciences Press.

Brody, E. (1981). "Women in the middle" and family help to older people. *The Gerontologist, 21,* 471–480.

Brody, S. J., Poulshock, S., & Masciocchi, C. (1978). The family caring unit: A major consideration in the long-term support system. *The Gerontologist, 18,* 556–561.

Brotman, H. B. (1977). Population projections: Part 1, Tomorrow's older population (to 2000). *The Gerontologist, 17,* 203–209.

Brown, C. (1984). *The art of coalition building: A guide for community leaders.* New York: The American Jewish Committee.

Buber, M. (1976). *The way of man according to the teaching of Hasidism.* Secaucus, NJ: The Citadel Press.

Butler, R. N., & Lewis, M. I. (1982). *Aging and mental health: Positive psychosocial and biomedical approaches* (3rd ed.). St. Louis: Mosby.

Cantor, M. H. (1976). Effect of ethnicity on life styles of the inner-city elderly. In A. Monk (Ed.), *The age of aging: A reader in social gerontology* (pp. 241–264). Buffalo, NY: Prometheus Books.

Cantor, M. H. (1979). The informal support system of New York's inner city elderly: Is ethnicity a factor? In D. E. Gelfand & A. J. Kutzik (Eds.), *Ethnicity and aging: Theory, research, and policy* (pp. 153–174). New York: Springer.

Cantor, M. H. (1983). Strain among caregivers: A study of experiences in the United States. *The Gerontologist, 23,* 597–604.

Carp, F. M., & Kataoka, E. (1976). Health care problems of the elderly of San Francisco's Chinatown. *The Gerontologist, 16*, 30–38.

The Catholic University of America, The Center for the Study of Pre-Retirement and Aging. (1979, November 15). *Symposium on older Americans of Euro-ethnic origin.* Washington, DC: Author.

Chen, P. N. (1979). A study of Chinese-American elderly residing in hotel rooms. *Social Casework: The Journal of Contemporary Social Work, 60*, 89–93.

Chrisman, N. J., & Kleinman, A. (1980). Health beliefs and practices. In S. T. Thernstrom, A. Orlov, & O. Handlin (Eds.), *Harvard encyclopedia of American ethnic groups* (pp. 452–462). Cambridge, MA: Belknap Press of Harvard University Press.

Clark, M., & Anderson, B. G. (1967). *Culture and aging.* Springfield, IL: Charles C. Thomas.

Cohler, B., & Grunebaum, H. (1981). *Mothers and daughters: Personality and childcare in three generation families.* New York: John Wiley.

Cohler, B., Lieberman, M., & Welch, L. (1976). *Social relations and interpersonal relations among middle-aged and older Irish, Italian, and Polish-American men and women.* Unpublished manuscript.

Colen, J. N., & Soto, D. (1979). *Service delivery to aged minorities: Techniques of successful programs.* Sacramento, CA: California State University, School of Social Work.

Comptroller General of the United States. (1977a). *Home health—the need for a national policy to better provide for the elderly.* Washington, DC: U.S. General Accounting Office.

Comptroller General of the United States. (1977b). *The well-being of older people in Cleveland, Ohio.* Washington: U.S. General Accounting Office.

Conzen, K. N. (1980). Germans. In S. T. Thernstrom, A. Orlov, & O. Handlin (Eds.), *Harvard encyclopedia of American ethnic groups* (pp. 405–425). Cambridge, MA: Belknap Press of Harvard University Press.

Cox, C., & Gelfand, D. (1985, November). *Patterns of family assistance, exchange, and filial satisfaction among ethnic elderly.* Paper presented at the meetings of the Gerontological Society of America, New Orleans.

Crandall, R. C. (1980). *Gerontology, a behavioral science approach.* Reading, MA: Addison-Wesley.

Creedon, M. A. (1985, May 17–18). *The role of the church/synagogue ministry in the lives of Euro-American elderly and their families.* Paper presented at the National Conference on Euro-American Elderly, The Catholic University of America, Washington, DC.

Creedon, M. A. (in preparation). Perspectives of pastors on services to the elderly in Euro-American parishes.

Croats. (1980). In S. T. Thernstrom, A. Orlov, & O. Handlin (Eds.), *Harvard encyclopedia of American ethnic groups* (pp. 247–252). Cambridge, MA: Belknap Press of Harvard University Press.

Cronin, C. (1970). *Sting of change: Sicilians in Sicily and Australia.* Chicago: University of Chicago Press.

Cuellar, J., Stanford, E. P., & Miller-Soule, D. I. (Eds.). (1982). *Understanding minority aging. Perspectives and sources.* San Diego, CA: San Diego State University Press.

Doty, P., Liu, K., & Wiener, Y. (1985). An overview of long-term care. *Health Care Financing Review, 6,* 69–78.

Dunlop, B. D. (1980). Expanded home-based care for the impaired elderly: Solution or pipe dream? *American Journal of Public Health, 70,* 514–519.

Ehrlich, P. (1979, December). *The mutual help model: Handbook for developing a neighborhood group program.* Washington, DC: Department of Health, Education & Welfare, Administration on Aging.

Eribes, A., & Bradley-Rawls, M. (1978). The underutilization of nursing home facilities by Mexican-American elderly in the Southwest. *The Gerontologist, 18,* 363–371.

Erickson, F. (1975). Gatekeeping and the melting pot: Interaction in counseling encounters. *Harvard Educational Review, 45,* 1, 44–70.

Erikson, E. H. (1963). *Childhood and society.* New York: W. W. Norton.

Erikson, E. H. (1968). *Identity, youth, and crisis.* New York: W. W. Norton.

Estes, C. (1979). *The aging enterprise.* San Francisco: Jossey-Bass.

Fandetti, D. V. (1974). *Sources of assistance in a white working class neighborhood.* Unpublished Ph.D. dissertation, Columbia University, New York.

Fandetti, D. V., & Gelfand, D. E. (1976). Care of the aged: Attitudes of white ethnic families. *The Gerontologist, 16,* 544–549.

Fecher, J. V. (1982). *Religion and aging, an annotated bibliography.* San Antonio, TX: Trinity University Press.

Federal Council on the Aging. (1976). *Annual report to the President, 1976.* Washington, DC: U.S. Government Printing Office.

Federal Register, September 4, 1985.

Finney, J. M., & Lee, G. R. (1977). Age differences on five dimensions of religious involvement. *Review of Religious Research, 18*(2), 173–179.

Fishman, J. A. (1966). *Language loyalty in the United States: The maintenance and perpetuation of non-English mother tongues by American ethnic and religious groups.* London: Mouton.

Fishman, J. A. (1980). Language maintenance. In S. T. Thernstrom, A. Orlov, & O. Handlin (Eds.), *Harvard encyclopedia of American ethnic groups* (pp. 629–638). Cambridge, MA: The Belknap Press of Harvard University Press.

Fishman, J. A. (1981). Language policy: Past, present, and future. In C. A. Ferguson & S. B. Heath (Eds.), *Language in the U.S.A.* (pp. 516–526). Cambridge, England: Cambridge University Press.

Fitzpatrick, K., & Logan, J. (1985). The aging of the suburbs, 1960–1980. *American Sociological Review, 50,* 106–116.

Frank, B. (1980). The American Orthodox Jewish grandmother: Ethnic change and stability. In A. Bloom (Ed.), *Selected studies on aging research in the social sciences at the graduate school and university center of the City University of New York* (pp. 64–69). (ERIC Document Reproduction Service No. ED 194 854)

Frankfather, D., Smith, M., & Capers, O. (1979, April). *Family maintenance of the disabled elderly.* Paper presented at the meeting of the American Orthopsychiatric Association, Washington, DC.

Freeze, K. J. (1980). Czechs. In S. T. Thernstrom, A. Orlov, & O. Handlin (Eds.), *Harvard encyclopedia of American ethnic groups* (pp. 261–272). Cambridge, MA: Belknap Press of Harvard University Press.

Froland, C., Pancoast, D. L., Chapman, N. J., & Kimboko, P. J. (1981). *Helping networks and human services.* Beverly Hills, CA: Sage Publications.

Fujii, S. M. (1976). Elderly Asian Americans and use of public services. *Social Casework, 57,* 202–207.

Gans, H. H. (1962). *The urban villagers.* New York: Free Press.

Gelfand, D. E. (1982). Aging: The ethnic factor. Boston: Little, Brown.

Gelfand, D. E. (1984). *The aging network: Programs and services* (2nd ed.). New York: Springer.

Gelfand, D. E. (in press). Assisting the new Russian elderly. *The Gerontologist.*

Gelfand, D. E., & Fandetti, D. V. (1980). Suburban and urban white ethnics: Attitudes towards care of the elderly. *The Gerontologist, 20,* 588–594.

Gelfand, D. E., Olsen, J., & Block, M. (1978). Two generations of elderly in the changing American family. *The Family Coordinator, 27,* 395–404.

Gelman, D., Hager, M., Gonzalez, D., Morris, H., McCormick, J., Jackson, T., & Karagianis, E. (1985, May 6). Who's taking care of our parents? *Newsweek,* pp. 60–73.

General Assembly of Pennsylvania. (1985 session). Senate Bill, No. 1107. Harrisburg: Author.

Gerber, L. (1983). Ethnicity still matters: Socio-demographic profiles of the ethnic elderly in Ontario. *Canadian Ethnic Studies, 15,* 60–80.

The Gerontological Society of America. Statement of the Gerontological Society of America (1985, February 21). Prepared for panel on Tomorrow's Elderly for the Congressional Clearinghouse on the Future (Draft). Washington, DC: Author.

Giordano, J. (1973). *Ethnicity and mental health research and recommendations.* New York: Institute on Pluralism and Group Identity.

Giordano, J., & Giordano, G. P. (1976, May/June). Ethnicity and community mental health: A review of the literature. *Community Mental Health Review, 1,* 3.

Giordano, J., & Levine, I. M. (1984). *Ethnicity and aging.* Report submitted to the New York City Department of Aging. New York: The American Jewish Committee, Institute of Human Relations.

Glazer, N. (1971). The limits of social policy. *Commentary, 52,* 51–58.

Glazer, N. (1984, October–November). The structure of ethnicity. *Public Opinion,* pp. 2–5.

Glazer, N., & Moynihan, D. P. (1970). *Beyond the melting pot* (2nd ed.). Cambridge, MA: Massachusetts Institute of Technology Press.

Gleason, P. (1980). American identity and Americanization. In S. T. Thernstrom, A. Orlov, & O. Handlin (Eds.), *Harvard encyclopedia of American ethnic groups* (pp. 31–58). Cambridge, MA: Belknap Press of Harvard University Press.

Glock, C. Y., & Stark, R. (1965). *Religion and society in tension.* Chicago: Rand McNally.

Goren, A. A. (1980). Jews. In S. T. Thernstrom, A. Orlov, & O. Handlin (Eds.), *Harvard encyclopedia of American ethnic groups* (pp. 571–598). Cambridge, MA: Belknap Press of Harvard University Press.

Greeley, A. (1972). *That most distressful nation.* Chicago: Quadrangle Books.

Greene, V. (1980). Poles. In S. T. Thernstrom, A. Orlov, & O. Handlin (Eds.), *Harvard encyclopedia of American ethnic groups* (pp. 787–803). Cambridge, MA: Belknap Press of Harvard University Press.

Gutman, D. L. (1966). *Work, culture, and society in industrializing America.* New York: Knopf.

Guttmann, D. (1973). Leisure time activity interests of Jewish aged. *The Gerontologist, 13,* 2.

Guttmann, D., Kolm, R., Mostwin, D., Kestenbaum, S., Harrington, D., Mullaney, J. W., Adams, K., Suziedelis, G., & Varga, L. (1979a). *Informal and formal support systems and their effect on the lives of the elderly in selected ethnic groups.* (Final report, Administration on Aging Grant No. 90-A-1007.) Washington, DC: National Catholic School of Social Service, The Catholic University of America.

Guttmann, D., Kolm, R., Mostwin, D., Kestenbaum, S., Harrington, D., Mullaney, J. W., Adams, K., Suziedelis, G., & Varga, L. (1979b). Use of informal and formal supports by white ethnic aged. In D. Gelfand & A. J. Kutzik (Eds.), *Ethnicity and aging: Theory, research, and policy* (pp. 246–262). New York: Springer.

Habenstein, R. W., & Mindel, C. H. (1981). The American ethnic family: Protean and adaptive patterns. In C. H. Mindel & R. W. Habenstein, (Eds.), *Ethnic families in America: Patterns and variations* (2nd ed.) (pp. 417–432). New York: Elsevier.

Haber, D. (1983). Promoting mutual help groups among older persons. *The Gerontologist, 23,* 251–253.

Harel, Z., Luick, M., & Wyatt, J. (1983). *Older American service consumers in Western Reserve.* Cleveland, OH: Cleveland State University, Gerontological Studies Program.

Harel, Z., Noelker, L., & Blake, B. (1985). Planning services for the elderly: Theoretical and research perspectives. *The Gerontologist, 25*(6), 644–649.

Harel, Z., Wyatt, J., & Luick, M. (1984). Older Americans Act service consumers: A contrast between the homebound and users of nutrition programs. *Journal of Gerontological Social Work, 6*(4), 19–34.

Hareven, T., & Modell, J. (1980). Family patterns. In S. Thernstrom, A. Orlov, & O. Handlin (Eds.), *Harvard encyclopedia of American ethnic groups* (pp. 345–354). Cambridge, MA: Belknap Press of Harvard University Press.

Harris, L. & Associates, Inc. (1976). *The myth and reality of aging in America.* Washington, DC: National Council on Aging.

Hatch, E. M. (1983). *Psycholinguistics: A second language perspective* (pp. 188–197). Rowley, MA: Newbury House Publishers.

Heidelberger Forschungsprojekt. (1978). The acquisition of German syntax by foreign migrant workers. In D. Sankoff (Ed.), *Linguistic variation: Model and methods* (pp. 1–22). New York: Academic Press.

Higham, J. (1980). Leadership. In S. T. Thernstrom, A. Orlov, & O. Handlin (Eds.), *Harvard encyclopedia of American ethnic groups* (pp. 642–647). Cambridge, MA: Belknap Press of Harvard University Press.

Hill, J. H. (1970). Foreign accents, language learning, cerebral dominance revisited. *Language Learning, 20,* 237–248.

Holmes, L. D. (1983). *Other cultures, elder years: An introduction to cultural gerontology.* Minneapolis, MN: Burgess.

Holzberg, C. S. (1982). Ethnicity and aging: Anthropological perspectives on more than just the minority elderly. *The Gerontologist, 22,* 249–257.

Howe, I. (1976). *World of our fathers.* New York: Harcourt, Brace, Jovanovich.

Hunter, C., & Harman, D. D. (1985 edition). *Adult illiteracy in the United States: A report to the Ford Foundation.* New York: McGraw Hill.

Huntington, G. E. (1981). The Amish family. In C. H. Mindel & R. W. Habenstein (Eds.), *Ethnic families in America* (pp. 295–322). New York: Elsevier.

Huttman, E. (1985). *Social services for the elderly.* New York: Free Press.

Huyck, M. H., & Hoyer, W. J. (1982). *Adult development and aging.* Belmont, CA: Wadsworth.

Jackson, M., & Harel, Z. (1983). Ethnic differences in social support networks. *Urban Health, 12,* 35–38.

Johnson, C. (1985). *Growing up and growing old in Italian-American families.* New Brunswick, NJ: Rutgers University Press.

Johnson, C., & Catalano, D. (1983). A longitudinal study of family supports to impaired elderly. *The Gerontologist, 23,* 612–618.

Johnson, E. (1981). Dyadic family relations and social support. *International Journal of Aging and Human Development, 14,* 271–276.

Kahana, E., & Felton, B. (1977). Social context and personal need: A study of Polish and Jewish aged. *Journal of Social Issues, 33,* 56–64.

Kalish, R. A. (1979). The religious triad: Church, clergy, faith. *Generations, 3,* 27–28.

Kalish, R. A. (1983). *The psychology of human behavior* (5th ed.). Monterey, CA: Brooks/Cole.

Kalish, R. A., & Visher, E. (1981). Grandparents of divorce. *Journal of Divorce, 5,* 127–140.

Kandel, R. F. (1979). Friendship and factionalism in a tri-ethnic housing complex for the elderly in north Miami. *Anthropological Quarterly, 52,* 49–59.

Kane, R. A., & Kane, R. L. (1984). *Assessing the elderly.* Lexington, MA: Lexington Books.

Kart, C. S. (1985). *The realities of aging* (2nd ed.). Boston: Allyn & Bacon.

Katz, D., Gutch, B. A., Kahn, R. L., & Barton, L. (1975). *Bureaucratic encounters: A pilot study in the evaluation of government services.* Ann Arbor: University of Michigan, Survey Research Center, Institute of Social Research.

Kent, O., & Matson, M. (1972). The impact of health on the aged family. *Family Coordinator, 21,* 29–36.

Lowy, L. (1985). *Social work with the aging.* New York: Longman.

Luebke, F. C. (1980). Legal restrictions on foreign languages in the Great Plains States. In F. C. Luebke (Ed.), *Languages in conflict: Linguistic acculturation on the Great Plains* (pp. 1–20). Lincoln, NE: University of Nebraska Press.

Lurie, E. (1978, November). *Adjustment of older persons after acute hospitalization.* Paper presented at the annual meeting of the Gerontological Society of America, Dallas, TX.

Macías, R. F. (1979). Choice of language as a human right—public policy implications in the United States. In R. Padilla, *Ethnoperspectives in bilingual education research: Bilingual education and public policy in the United States* (pp. 39–57). Ypsilanti, MI: Eastern Michigan University.

Macías, R. F. (1984a). *Demystifying the concept of culture.* Unpublished manuscript.

Macías, R. F. (1984b). *Institutional languages policies: A medical and hospital services case study.* Unpublished manuscript.

Magocsi, P. R. (1980). Ukrainians. In S. T. Thernstrom, A. Orlov, & O. Handlin (Eds.), *Harvard encyclopedia of American ethnic groups* (pp. 997–1009). Cambridge, MA: Belknap Press of Harvard University Press.

Markides, K. S. (1982). Ethnicity and aging: A comment. *The Gerontologist, 11,* 467–470.

Markson, E. W. (1979). Ethnicity as a factor in the institutionalization of the ethnic elderly. In D. E. Gelfand & A. J. Kutzik (Eds.), *Ethnicity and aging: Theory, research and policy* (pp. 341–356). New York: Springer.

Maslow, A. H. (1970). *Motivation and personality* (2nd ed.). New York: Harper & Row.

Mathias, C. (1981, Summer). *Foreign Affairs, 59,* pp. 975–998.

Maves, P. B., & Cedarleaf, J. L. (1949). *Older people and the church.* New York: Abingdon-Cokesbury Press.

McCourt, K. (1979). Euro-ethnic women: Some observations. *The Euro-ethnic Americans in the U.S.* Paper presented at the U.S. Civil Rights Commission Hearing, Chicago.

McMullin, M. (1985, April). Interview on the Greek American community, conducted in Long Beach, CA.

Mindel, C. H., & Habenstein, R. W. (1976). *Ethnic families in America.* New York: Elsevier.

Minkler, M., & Stone, R. (1985). The feminization of poverty and older women. *The Gerontologist, 25,* 351–357.

Moberg, D. O. (1971). *Spiritual well-being.* (White House Conference on Aging background paper). Washington, DC: U.S. Government Printing Office.

Moberg, D. O. (1983). The ecological fallacy: Concerns for program planners. *Generations, 8*(1), 12–14.

Moore, J. (1976). Situational factors affecting minority aging. In B. Bell (Ed.), *Contemporary social gerontology.* Springfield, IL: C. C. Thomas.

Mostwin, D. (1979). Emotional needs of elderly Americans of central and eastern European background. In D. E. Gelfand & A. J. Kutzik (Eds.), *Ethnicity and aging: Theory, research, and policy* (pp. 263–276). New York: Springer.

Murguia, E., Schultz, T. M., Markides, K. S., & Janson, P. (1984). *Ethnicity and aging: A bibliography.* San Antonio, TX: Trinity University Press.

Murray, H. A. (1938). *Explorations in personality.* New York: Oxford University Press.

Naparstek, A., Biegel, D., & Spence, B. (1978). *Neighborhood and family services project community analysis data report* (Vol. 1). Washington, DC: University of Southern California Washington Public Affairs Center.

National Center for Health Statistics. (1972). Home care for persons 65 and over, U.S., July 1966–June 1968. In *Vital Health Statistics,* Series No. 73. Washington, DC: Department of Health and Welfare Publications, HSM72-1062.

National Conference on Social Welfare. (1977). *The future for social welfare in the United States.* Final report of the task force on the organization and delivery of human services: The public, private, and consumer partnership. Washington, DC: Author.

National Council on the Aging. (1981). Local coalition: Cooperation and coordination between senior centers and other aging service providers. *Senior Center Report, 4*(5), 2, 5–6.

Nelli, H. S. (1980). Italians. In S. T. Thernstrom, A. Orlov, & O. Handlin (Eds.), *Harvard encyclopedia of American ethnic groups* (pp. 545–560). Cambridge, MA: Belknap Press of Harvard University Press.

Neugarten, Bernice L. (1974). Age groups in American society and the rise of the young-old. *Annals of the American Academy of Political and Social Sciences, 415,* 187–198.

New York Times. (July 22, 1985). Style.

Noelker, L., & Poulshock, W. (1982). *The effects on families of caring for impaired elderly in residence.* Cleveland, OH: The Benjamin Rose Institute.

Older Americans Act, Amended, 1965. (1985). (Sections: 305 (a)(2)(E) Organization; 307 (a)(13) State Plans; 305 (d)(2); 306 (a)(5)(A); 422 (b)(6); 502 (c)(M). P.L. 98-459 dated October 7, 1984, 55 pp.) Washington, DC: U.S. Government Printing Office.

Olneck, M. R., & Lazerson, M. (1980). Education. In S. T. Thernstrom, A. Orlov, & O. Handlin (Eds.), *Harvard encyclopedia of American ethnic groups* (pp. 303–319). Cambridge, MA: Belknap Press of Harvard University Press.

Oxford, R. L. (1980, September 30). Projections of the number of limited English proficient (LEP) persons to the year 2000. Final report, Inter-America Research Associates, Inc. Submitted to the National Center for Educational Statistics, Los Angeles.

Parsons, T. (1968). *The social system.* New York: Free Press.

Pasquariello, R. P. (1979). *Like the fingers of the hand: Religion and ethnicity in the Italian-American experience.* (Presentation to the Trinity College Theology Society). Washington, DC: Trinity College.

Peralta, V., & Horikawa, H. (1978). *Needs and potentialities assessment of Asian-American elderly in greater Philadelphia.* (ERIC Document Reproduction Service No. ED 167 661).

Perdue, C. (Ed.). (1984). *Second language acquisition by adult immigrants: A field manual.* Rowley, MA: Newbury House.

Petersen, W. (1985, Summer). Defining Americans. *The Wilson Quarterly,* pp. 97 ff.

Petersen, W., Novak, M., & Gleason, P. (1982). *Concepts of ethnicity.* In S. T. Thernstrom, A. Orlov, & O. Handlin (Eds.), *Harvard encyclopedia of American ethnic groups* (pp. 234–242). Cambridge, MA: The Belknap Press of Harvard University Press.

Petrovich, M. B., & Halpern, J. (1980). Serbs. In S. T. Thernstrom, A. Orlov, & O. Handlin (Eds.), *Harvard encyclopedia of American ethnic groups* (pp. 916–926). Cambridge, MA: Belknap Press of Harvard University Press.

Pitt, L. (1976). *We Americans: A topical history of the United States: Vol. 1, Colonial Times to 1877.* Glenview, IL: Scott, Foresman.

Powers, E., & Bultena, G. (1974). Correspondence between anticipated and actual use of public services by the aged. *Social Service Review, 48,* 245–254.

President's Commission on Mental Health. (1978). *Special populations* (Vol. 3, Appendix). Washington, DC: U.S. Government Printing Office 276-135/6522.

Price, C. A. (1980). Methods of estimating the size of groups (Appendix). In S. T. Thernstrom, A. Orlov, & O. Handlin (Eds.), *Harvard encyclopedia of American ethnic groups* (pp. 1033–1044). Cambridge: Belknap Press of Harvard University Press.

Princeton Religion Research Center. (1982). *Religion in America, 1982.* Princeton, NJ: The Gallup Poll.

Quam, J. (1984). National helpers: Tools for working with the chronically mentally ill elderly. *The Gerontologist, 24*(6), 564–567.

Rogers, F. (1980). In S. T. Thernstrom, A. Orlov, & O. Handlin (Eds.), *Harvard encyclopedia of American ethnic groups* (pp. 813–820). Cambridge, MA: Belknap Press of Harvard University Press.

Rosow, I. (1967). *Social integration of the aged.* New York: Free Press.

Ross, J. K. (1977). *Old people, new lives.* Chicago: University of Chicago Press.

Rowan, C. (August 26, 1981). New poverty figures mean new trouble. *Washington Post.*

Ruffini, J. L., & Todd, H. F. (1979). A network model for leadership development among the elderly. *The Gerontologist, 19,* 150–162.

Saloutos, T. (1980). Greeks. In S. T. Thernstrom, A. Orlov, & O. Handlin (Eds.), *Harvard encyclopedia of American ethnic groups* (pp. 430–440). Cambridge, MA: Belknap Press of Harvard University Press.

Sauer, W. J., & Coward, R. T. (1985). *Social support networks and the care of the elderly.* New York: Springer.

Saville-Troike, M. (1978). *A guide to culture in the classroom.* Rosslyn, VA: National Clearinghouse for Bilingual Education.

Schaie, K. W., & Geiwitz, J. (1982). *Adult development and aging.* Boston: Little, Brown.

Schooler, C. (1976). Serfdom's legacy: An ethnic continuum. *American Journal of Sociology, 81,* 1265–1285.

Shanas, E. (1979). Social myth as hypothesis: The case of family relations of older people. *The Gerontologist, 19,* 3–9.

Sheehan, S. (1984). *Kate Quinton's days.* New York: Houghton-Mifflin.

Silverstein, N. (1984). Informing the elderly about public services: The relationship between sources of knowledge and service utilization. *The Gerontologist, 24,* 37–40.

Simon, P. (1980). *The tongue-tied American: Confronting the foreign language crisis.* New York: Continuum.

Simos, B. (1973). Adult children and their aging parents. *Social Work, 18,* 75–85.

Skårdal, D. B. (1980). Danes. In S. T. Thernstrom, A. Orlov, & O. Handlin (Eds.), *Harvard encyclopedia of American ethnic groups* (pp. 273–281). Cambridge, MA: Belknap Press of Harvard University Press.

Soldo, B. J. (1980). America's elderly in the 1980s. *Population Bulletin, 35*(4). Washington, DC: Population Reference Bureau, Inc.

Spicer, E. H. (1981). *Cycles of conquest.* Tucson, AZ: University of Arizona Press.

Spiegel, J., & Papajohn, J. (1983, July). *Final report of training programs in ethnicity and mental health.* (NIMH Grant MH #5-T24-Mh 14962). Washington, DC: National Institutes of Mental Health.

Stanford, E. P. (1978). The ethnic elders. San Diego, CA: San Diego State University.

Stanford, E. P. (Ed). (1979). *Minority aging research: Old issues—new approaches.* San Diego, CA: University of San Diego.

Staples, R. (1976). *Introduction to black sociology.* New York: McGraw-Hill.

Sterne, R. S., Phillips, J. E., & Rabushka, A. (1974). *The urban elderly poor.* Lexington, MA: Lexington Books.

Stolarik, M. M. (1980). Slovaks. In S. T. Thernstrom, A. Orlov, & O. Handlin (Eds.), *Harvard encyclopedia of American ethnic groups* (pp. 926–934). Cambridge, MA: Belknap Press of Harvard University Press.

Struening, E., Rabkin, K., & Peck, H. (1970). Migration and ethnic membership in relation to social problems. In R. Brody (Ed.), *Behavior in new environments.* Beverly Hills, CA: Sage.

Stuen, C. (1985). Community organization. In A. Monk (Ed.), *Handbook of gerontological services.* New York: Van Nostrand Reinhold.

Sussman, M. B. (1979, January). *Social and economic supports and family environments for the elderly.* (Final Report to the Administration on Aging). Washington, DC: Administration on Aging.

Taylor, B. P. (1974). Toward a theory of language acquisition. *Language Learning, 24*(1), 23–35.

Thernstrom, S. T., Orlov, A., & Handlin, O. (Eds.). (1980). *Harvard encyclopedia of American ethnic groups.* Cambridge, MA: Belknap Press of Harvard University Press.

Tobin, S., & Ellor, J. (1983). The church and the aging network: More interaction needed. *Generations, 8*(1), 26–29.

Torres-Gil, F. (1983). Political involvement among older members of national minority groups: Problems and prospects. In R. L. McNeely and J. L. Cohen

(Eds.), *Aging in Minority Groups* (pp. 226–236). Beverly Hills, CA: Sage Publications.

Towle, C. (1952). *Common human needs.* New York: American Association of Social Workers.

Ujvagi, P. (1979). Response. In *A consultation on civil rights issues of Euro-ethnic Americans in the U.S.: Opportunities and challenges* (pp. 192–198). Chicago: U.S. Civil Rights Commission.

U.S. Bureau of the Census. (1983). Ancestry of the population by state: 1980. *Supplementary report of the 1980 census of population.* (PC80-S1-10). Washington, DC: Author.

U.S. Bureau of the Census (1984, October 7). Socioeconomic characteristics of U.S. foreign-born population. Detailed in Census Bureau tabulations, *U.S. Department of Commerce News.* Washington, DC: Author.

U.S. Civil Rights Commission. (1979, December 3). *A consultation on civil rights issues of Euro-ethnic Americans in the U.S.: Opportunities and challenges.* Chicago: Author.

U.S. Civil Rights Commission. (1982). *Minority elderly services: New programs, old problems* (Part 1). Chicago: Author.

U.S. Conference of Mayors. (1982). *Administering aging programs: Coordinating services for the urban elderly.* (Prepared under a grant from the Administration on Aging, 90-AM-5/02.) Washington, DC: U.S. Department of Health and Human Services.

U.S. Congress, 92nd Cong. P.L. 92-258.

U.S. Congress. House Select Committee on Children, Youth, and Families (1984). *Demographic and social trends: Implications for federal support of dependent-care services for children and the elderly.* Washington, DC: U.S. Government Printing Office (28-767-0).

U.S. Congress. Senate. Special Committee on Aging. (1984). *Developments in aging.* Washington, DC: U.S. Government Printing Office.

U.S. Department of Health and Human Services. Office for Civil Rights, Region X. (1985). *How to establish effective communication procedures for persons with limited English proficiency and for persons with impaired hearing, vision, or speech.* Seattle, WA: Author.

U.S. Health Services Administration. (1973). *Home health in Chinatown.* Washington, DC: U.S. Government Printing Office.

Veltman, C. (1983). *Language shift in the United States.* New York: Mouton.

Watson, W. H. (1982). *Aging and social behavior—an introduction to social gerontology.* Monterey, CA: Wadsworth Health Sciences Division.

Webster's new ideal dictionary. (1978). Springfield, MA: G. L. C. Merriam.

White House Conference on Aging. (1981). *Final Report* (Vol. 1). Washington, DC: U.S. Government Printing Office.

White House Conference on Aging. (1981). *Report of the Mini-Conference on Euro-American Elderly, November 10–12, 1980.* Baltimore: Author.

Wright, J. D., Rossi, P. H., & Juravich, T. F. (1980). Survey Research. In S. T. Thernstrom, A. Orlov, & O. Handlin (Eds.), *Harvard encyclopedia of American ethnic groups* (pp. 951–971). Cambridge, MA: Belknap Press of Harvard University Press.

Author Index

Subject Index